Ethics and the Metaphysics of Medicine

Basic Bioethics
Glenn McGee and Arthur Caplan, editors

Ethics and the Metaphysics of Medicine

Reflections on Health and Beneficence

Kenneth A. Richman

The MIT Press
Cambridge, Massachusetts
London, England

This book was set in Sabon by SNP Best-set Typesetter Ltd., Hong Kong.

Printed and bound in the United States of America.

Library of Congress Cataloging-in-Publication Data

Ethics and the metaphysics of medicine : reflections on health and beneficence / Kenneth A. Richman, [editor].
    p. cm.—(Basic bioethics)
Includes bibliographical references and index.
ISBN 0-262-18238-6 (hc : alk. paper)
1. Medicine—Philosophy 2. Health—Philosophy. 3. Medical ethics.
4. Hume, David, 1711–1776. I. Richman, Kenneth A., 1966– II. Title.
III. Series.

R723.N4427   2004
610′.1—dc22

                                                      2003068567

10   9   8   7   6   5   4   3   2   1

Contents

Series Foreword

We are pleased to present the eleventh book in the series Basic Bioethics. The series presents innovative works in bioethics to a broad audience and introduces seminal scholarly manuscripts, state-of-the-art reference works, and textbooks. Such broad areas as the philosophy of medicine, advancing genetics and biotechnology, end of life care, health and social policy, and the empirical study of biomedical life are engaged.

Glenn McGee
Arthur Caplan

Basic Bioethics Series Editorial Board
Tod S. Chambers
Susan Dorr Goold
Mark Kuczewski
Herman Saatkamp

Preface and Acknowledgments

Acquaintances occasionally ask how I ended up working on the philosophy of medicine after writing a dissertation on the history of eighteenth-century philosophy, and are surprised to hear that my work on health arose directly from my work on David Hume's theory of belief. To argue that Hume valued certain beliefs because of their status as components of the mental life of healthy, well-functioning humans, I began to think about what it means to be a healthy individual. I eventually drafted a short paper on concepts of health for a conference and sent it to some of the more philosophically minded physicians I know. Andrew Budson, an old friend from our undergraduate days at Haverford, where philosophy seems to matter more than at most places, telephoned full of questions and objections. Always thinking, my wife Leslie suggested the collaboration that resulted in what I call the Richman–Budson theory of health.

This theory is developed, expanded, and defended in part I of this book. The remaining parts explore its practical and ethical implications. The topics covered range from the philosophy of science to Kantian ethics to knee surgery. Although the treatment is technical, academic philosophy, I hope to have shown something of the contribution that the more theoretical aspects of philosophy can make to the daily lives of individuals and communities.

In addition to Andrew Budson and Leslie Anne Richman, many people have supported this project in many ways. I am indebted to Ronald Munson for taking time to read the early chapters and offer comments and kind words, and to Aaron T. Beck for helpful thoughts on cognitive therapy and health. I am grateful for financial support from Bryn Mawr

College, from the Kalamazoo College Faculty Development Committee, and from the Paul Todd Sr. Endowment for Philosophy at Kalamazoo College. Kluwer Academic Publishers kindly granted permission for use of material originally appearing in my article with Andrew Budson in *Theoretical Medicine and Bioethics*. Students in my Philosophy of Medicine course at Bryn Mawr College helped me to develop my thoughts and explanations, as did the several Matts and other philosophy students at K College.

Among many others, I thank the individuals listed below. In acknowledging their encouragement, input, and support, I in no way wish to taint them with any infelicities of style or content to be found herein.

The Fellows and staff of the University of Pennsylvania Center for Bioethics, especially Art Caplan, David Doukas, David Magnus, and Dominic Sisti

Martha Brandt Bolton, Philosophy, Rutgers University

Martin Bunzl, Philosophy, Rutgers University

Steven Frye, Librarian, University of Wisconsin

Paul Grobstein, Biology, Bryn Mawr College

Douglas Husak, Law and Philosophy, Rutgers University

Jodi Jacoby, Humanities Secretary, Bryn Mawr College

Peter Kivy, Philosophy, Rutgers University

Michael Krausz, Philosophy, Bryn Mawr College

Christopher Latiolais, Philosophy, Kalamazoo College

Susan S. Levine, LCSW

Clay Morgan, MIT Press

Joseph Rucker, Chemistry, Villanova University

Anne Sclufer, MSS, PhD

John Alexander

I
Theories of Health

1

The Question of Normativity

Definitions of health and disease, rather than being of academic use only, are critically important in our society. For instance, as there is currently no single standard of health care in the United States, the movement to define certain basic rights to health care is growing. Legislation such as the Patients' Bill of Rights is the result of this movement. Although few would argue against the desirability of childhood vaccinations or the right of a trauma victim to receive emergency medical care, it becomes less clear whether patients have "rights" to receive treatment for learning disabilities or for infertility. Indeed, it is a contentious issue whether such individuals have truly medical problems at all, or simply problems. Consider also our country's anti-discrimination laws, such as the Americans with Disabilities Act, which provides an individual with "a physical or mental impairment that substantially limits one or more of the major life activities of such individual" (1990, §12102) protection against discrimination on the basis of the disability. Legislators endeavored to state precisely what conditions should and should not be protected. Given that a number of exceptions had to be written in specifically, however, it is evident that they were unable to define "physical and mental impairments" and "major life activities" adequately. For example, a section of the Americans with Disabilities Act was included entirely to ensure that "disability" would not apply to an individual "solely because that individual is a transvestite" (1990, §12208).

Our understanding of what it means to be healthy is thus central to any number of issues, from doctor's notes presented to teachers and employers to the most wide-reaching legal matters. For instance, many people consider the health of a pregnant woman relevant to the abortion issue, claiming that abortion is permissible in cases where her health would be endangered by continuing the pregnancy.

In *Roe v. Wade*, Justice Blackmun delivered the opinion of the court:

... the State retains a definite interest in protecting the woman's own health and safety when an abortion is proposed at a late stage of pregnancy. (*Roe v. Wade* 1973, 174)

Blackmun held that changes in the state of medical knowledge and procedures can be relevant to whether abortion ought to be allowed insofar as they affect the expected impact on the woman's health (and safety). He took care to note that the woman's mental health is a factor, and not just her physical health, writing, "Mental and physical health may be taxed by child care" (*Roe v. Wade* 1973, 177).

It is remarkable that this opinion is presented in the complete absence of a theory of health. Blackmun stated that maintaining the health of women is in the interest of the state, but offered no guidance as to how we might go about determining when that health is endangered or compromised. Clearly, a richer understanding of the scope of terms such as "physical and mental impairments," "major life activities," "health," and "disease" can help us to create more consistent definitions and policies that in turn will help to understand and protect the rights of individuals and provide for a more just society.

This book is about the philosophy of medicine. Part I presents a theory of health, which makes it a study in metaphysics and the philosophy of science. Later parts are about the ethical implications of the theory defended in part I. This approach comes from the realization that knowing what it means for a person to be healthy is relevant to almost every medical encounter, and that clearer understanding of the goals of health care would allow professionals and patients to act more confidently and more responsibly. The conceit is that in order to improve the health of patients and populations, health care professionals and the patients themselves must be more thoughtful about *what health is*. The nature of health is a metaphysical issue central to the philosophy of medical science.

I take it as given that we have a concept of health, however rough, that we apply in our everyday interactions with the world and with one another. Although we may not have a definition that satisfies the standards of philosophy, we do have intuitions about what are healthy and unhealthy states. What we are looking for is an appropriate analysis of this concept, one that we will find enlightening and will, in general, be in accord with our intuitions. Of course, such an analysis may lead us to change our minds about things, and we may find ourselves with some new ideas. The goal is not, however, to replace our ordinary notion of health with something neat but foreign. It would do us no good to clarify what we mean when we talk about health in such a way that we end up with a completely different concept altogether. Our analysis must result in something that accords with the intuitions we hold most central or offer clear reasons for changing these intuitions. Furthermore, I will assume that if two people disagree on whether a given state is healthy, our analysis will either tell us that at least one of them is incorrect or give an account of how they can both be correct (in the way that ethical relativism gives an account of how people from different communities can disagree and both be correct about the moral value of some type of action).

A theory of health has crucial implications for the provision of medical care. Diagnosis, choosing among treatment options, outcomes assessment, and, of importance, how professionals talk to patients are all implicated. A theory of health can thus have an indirect effect on medical research as a result of changes in patterns of clinical diagnosis and treatment, and through changing patterns of requests from patients who begin to think of their own health differently. A theory can also have a direct impact on the course of research in medical science by shaping areas of investigation that are considered specifically health-related and hence medical.

Normativity and Medical Science

A fundamental feature of a theory of health is whether values play a role. Some theories tell us how things are and imply nothing about whether it is desirable that things be that way. Others tell us how things should be, are supposed to be, or ought to be; that is, how it is best for things to be. They identify certain states of affairs as having positive value, as being better than (at least some of) the alternatives. They are thus evaluative or, as I say, *normative*. For example, they tell us which states or conditions are healthy and that it is better to be in such a state or condition than not to be.

Another way of understanding this distinction is in terms of direction of fit. Descriptive theories are meant to conform to the facts. If the theories do not fit the facts, we blame the theories. Normative theories are such that the facts are supposed to fit them. If the facts do not fit the theories, we blame the facts. Thus, if an anthropologist offers a (descriptive) theory claiming that a culture with feature x must also have feature y when some cultures have x but not y, the anthropologist has a bad theory. But if the school dress code says that students are not to wear T-shirts, a student wearing a T-shirt shows not the code but himself to be bad. A key question for our project is whether health is a nonnormative or a normative concept.

Theorists such as Christopher Boorse, Arthur Caplan, and Thomas Szasz have suggested that normative theories are unscientific and without objective basis, and hence a normativist account of health will apply only within a particular culture and not universally.[1] To explain the nature of the debate over normativism in theories of health, Caplan (1993) wrote, "[t]he greater the role of values in the definition of health and disease, the worse the prognosis appears to be for both their objectivity and reality" (240–41). Issues that are a matter of value only, such as rules of etiquette, are said to be "merely" subjective, or conventional; they could be different without changes in the facts that science is interested in. Lack of consensus about issues concerning values, with etiquette and fashion perhaps the most compelling examples, looks like evidence that values lack the objectivity that would provide a basis for intersubjective agreement.

Szasz also acknowledged the important fact that people value health, while insisting that medical facts are just that—facts only, without normativity. These remarks came in the context of his famous position that mental illness is a dangerous myth of modern Western civilization. His primary reason for this position was captured as follows:

The norm from which deviation is measured whenever one speaks of a mental illness is a *psycho-social and ethical one*. Yet, the remedy is sought in terms of *medical* measures which—it is hoped and assumed—are free from wide differences of ethical value. (Szasz 1960, 114)

In short, Szasz believed that it is a mistake to address issues of value (such as, in his view, mental "health") with nonnormative tools of medical science. The assumption again is that where values exist, intersubjective agreement is not to be hoped for, and a realm in which intersubjective agreement cannot be hoped for is outside the scope of science and hence outside the scope of medicine.

Why do people insist that science is nonnormative? One reason is the tradition, stemming from Francis Bacon and others, of treating science as based entirely on observation. One can observe the way things are but not the way things ought to be. This connects with the familiar empiricist views of Locke, Berkeley, and Hume. It also connects with the empiricist tradition of logical positivism. Logical positivists such as A. J. Ayer went so far as to claim that statements regarding value, such as ethical and aesthetic judgments, were without cognitive meaning because they could not be verified by experience. All of this leads to the conclusion that if science is a possible object of knowledge, it does not involve normativity.

David Hume is particularly famous for drawing what we call "the fact-value distinction." In the famous "is–ought" passage of his *Treatise of Human Nature* (Hume 1978, 469), he objected to arguments with factual premises and normative conclusions. He claimed that it is "inconceivable" that a statement containing an "ought" or an "ought not" "can be a deduction from" statements containing only "is" or "is not." Hume is invoked by those who reject normativity in science. (However, the role of deduction in Hume's thinking is significant, and deduction is no longer a primary model for scientific reasoning.)

The view that science is strictly value neutral has serious implications. If we accept this view and we find that the correct understanding of health involves normativity, we may find ourselves stuck with the unwelcome conclusion that medical science (if it is to be understood as the scientific study of health) is not a science at all.[2]

A Philosophical Tale I: Is There a Difference between Biological and Physical Sciences?

In this section I will tell a philosopher's story about the sciences. I call it a philosopher's story because although I am quite attached to it, as are many of my philosophical acquaintances, it has been known to irritate scientists. Scientists looking at the first part of this story (the part told in this section) do not always find themselves reflected in it. I am going to tell it anyway because it will help us to understand some important features of medicine. Afterward I will backtrack a bit, attempting to hold onto the moral of the story even in the face of admitting that it was only a story.

Once upon a time, science was thought to be the reporting of objective, nonnormative fact. The intuition that science properly so called must be completely free of normativity has its roots in at least three traditional ways of thinking. One is the empiricist tradition noted above. Another is the tradition according to which scientific knowledge (*episteme* for Aristotle; *scientia* for Descartes) consists of either self-evident first principles or the conclusions of deductive arguments from such principles. According to this tradition, mathematics is the primary example of a science. The third is the tendency to see physics, specifically Newtonian mechanics, as nearly on a par with mathematics. The legitimacy of Newton's *Principia* in the seventeenth century lay in its presentation of a mathematical theory of motion.

Newtonian mechanics is characterized by laws that serve as first principles. These laws allow us to deduce with certainty facts about the mechanical properties of objects. Newton's laws of motion are successful because they do a good job of describing the way things actually are. They fit the facts. (For the purpose of our tale we will ignore the complications of modern physics.) Furthermore, they are quite specific. They do not give an *approximation* of the velocity to be expected in an object or a *range* into which we can expect it to fall. They do not indicate that an object "should" or "will usually" accelerate in a given way.

Biological sciences, including medical subfields, do not work this way. Generalizations of anatomy and physiology are not expected to hold strictly across all organisms. Instead, they offer a sort of idealized account of a "normal" subject. It is difficult to sort out what this means, as medical textbooks rarely address issues that concern philosophers of science. Instead, they tend to give average measurements and most common patterns and shapes (Basmajian and Slonecker 1989, xvii). Where they talk about extreme variations, they tend to use the terms "abnormality" and "anomaly":

Owing to the variety of these [measures and patterns], the commonest may have less than a 50% incidence; therefore, it may not be truly representative . . . Some variations are so rare as to be abnormalities or *anomalies*. (Basmajian and Slonecker 1989, xvii)

Here the authors of *Grant's Method of Anatomy* acknowledge that variations to be expected in anatomy are so great that there may not even *be* a representative structure.

Consider the following discussion of the skeletal system:

. . . it is often difficult to distinguish pathological from normal variation. Body height is an example: between the extremes of dwarfism and gigantism (both resulting from hormonal dysfunction), much variation in height occurs. (*Gray's Anatomy: The Anatomical Basis of Medicine and Surgery* 1995, 433)

Kenneth Lyons Jones discussed and categorized many ways in which humans can develop abnormally. Malformations are distinguished from deformations. Whereas deformations are "due to mechanical factors . . ." (Jones 1997, 1) impinging on development, many malformations are simply cases of things going wrong. Of course, many others are the predictable results of causes such as a woman's use of alcohol during pregnancy. However, even when the etiology of a malformation can be identified, we are told not to expect similar results in all similar cases. "Variance in extent of abnormality (expression) among individuals with the same etiologic syndrome is a usual phenomenon . . .", and "it is unusual to find a given anomaly in 100 per cent of patients with the same etiologic syndrome" (Jones 1997, 2–3).

'Anomalous' is used more or less interchangeably with 'abnormal.' (They differ slightly, as anomaly in these contexts seems to ring with its literal sense, indicating that a phenomenon falls outside the laws.) Two concepts of normality (and hence of abnormality) are found in medical texts, however, and most statements about normality in discussions of anatomy are ambiguous between them. One is the concept of statistical normality, which physicians use when they speak of a condition or state being normal *for a population*. This concept is not normative. It refers only to the range of states commonly found in a given population.

The other concept of normality is normative, and belongs to a family of related concepts, including health, disease, and proper functioning. This is the concept at work when physicians speak of what is normal *for an individual*. The structure or state that is normal for an individual allows that individual to function properly and thus maintain health. What is normal for an individual may be quite different from what is normal for the population of which that individual is a member.

According to my story, the fact that medical sciences allow for anomalies and abnormalities in the normative sense tells us a great deal about how these sciences differ from classical physics, and hence how the traditions identified at the beginning of this section can lead us to wonder whether medicine lives up to the standards of science properly so called. Because traditional science has at its core *laws*, part of these wonderings concern the status of the principles governing the medical sciences. Can principles allow for variations, even abnormalities and anomalies, and still be the principles or laws of a science?

Three sorts of scientific principles allow variation: probabilistic principles, ceteris paribus ("all things being equal") principles, and normative principles. All stand in contrast to the strict laws of Newtonian mechanics. Could the principles of anatomy be probabilistic laws? No, because the variations described by probabilistic laws are part of what the laws tell us to expect even when things are going in accordance with the laws. Different possible outcomes are equally predicted by probabilistic laws and explained by them. Consider the gambler's dice. Whereas some possible rolls are more desirable than others in the eyes of the gambler, they are equally good with respect to the laws of physics. In contrast, variations described by the anatomist are not predicted by principles. Medical abnormalities are evidence of something going wrong. Of course, because anatomical phenomena are also physical phenomena, there exists a level of description (biochemical, physical) at which laws cover and predict the anomaly. But at the level of description appropriate to their disciplines, an anatomist can find *mal*formations and a physiologist *mal*functions.

Could the principles of medical science be ceteris paribus laws, laws that hold not strictly or probabilistically but all things being equal? They are not ceteris paribus laws of the type that philosophers talk about today. A dominant view of ceteris paribus laws was proposed by Jerry Fodor in his discussion of the special sciences. Fodor spoke of laws in terms of subjunctive conditionals (counterfactuals), statements of the general form *if an event of type A occurs, then an event of type C occurs*. The types of events picked out by laws of a science are the types of events that are of interest to that science—the types of that science. The "if" clause of a conditional is called its *antecedent*; the "then" clause its *consequent*. In Fodor's picture, ceteris paribus laws of special sciences (psychology and the other sciences whose laws do not apply to everything in the world, unlike the laws of physics are supposed to) can have two types of exceptions. What he called "mere exceptions" occur because certain background or corollary conditions (called "completers") are not met.[3]

"Absolute exceptions" occur because the types that are picked out by laws of special sciences can be realized by states that fall into different types when described using the terms of a more basic science (generally, physics). This sort of "multiple realizability" is seen in the way that the same psychological events can be realized in different physical parts of the brain. For example, if parts of a young person's brain are removed to help the person avoid seizures, the capacity for language processing develops elsewhere. Because neurological development does not depend on location (anatomy), each event type studied by psychologists and neurologists can be realized by a variety of physical event types.

Most realizations of the special science type specified in the antecedent of the conditional stating the law will lead to the consequent of the law, which is what makes it a law. However, some realizations will not lead to realizations of the consequent, which is what makes it a ceteris paribus law. Realizations that constitute exceptions to this law count as realizations of the relevant special science type only if, for most laws of the special science involving that type, they are not exceptions.[4] So there is nothing less good about those realizations of the special science types that are absolute exceptions to a particular law, because with regard to other laws, they are not absolute exceptions, and other realizations that are not absolute exceptions to this law may be absolute exceptions to other laws.

Anatomy involves multiple realizability of normal states. For instance, a wide variety of different physical arrangements of blood vessels can count as normal. However, notions of malfunction and malformation carry evaluative vectors that are absent in exceptions to ceteris paribus laws.

Thus we are left with the conclusion that principles of medical science, allowing for variation in the specific way that they do, must be normative, with a direction of fit from facts to principles rather than vice versa. Of course, the variation is not just variation in how well an organism or part of an organism meets a normative standard. As noted in the anatomy texts cited, plenty of variation also exists among structures that do equally well at meeting a given standard. Eye color and precise placement of blood vessels are examples of this type of variation in the realm of multiple realizability.

A Philosophical Tale II: Normativity and Teleology

Our story has brought us back to values. "Normative science" is seen by many as an oxymoron because values will be relative and subjective, whereas science must (at least pretend to) be universal, absolute, and objective. So does the conclusion of the last section entail that medicine is not a science? I am not worried that normative principles are unscientific. Medicine is a biological science, and biology has some notions that are normative to some degree, such as the notion of proper functioning. I am also not worried that normativism necessarily entails relativism. If we can find an objective basis for normativity in health, we can have normativity and objectivity both. Our job in this section is to see how normativity fits into the biological sciences.

The sort of normativity we find in the biological sciences has to do with functions and goals. Colloquially, someone with malformed heart valves might say, "I have a bad ticker," and one with a permanent injury might explain a limp by referring to "my bum knee." These evaluative statements certainly tell us something about the speaker's relationship to these body parts; the body parts are not performing the function generally expected of them to the level hoped for by the person whose body parts they are. These statements have much in common with other evaluations of instrumental value, value relative to some goal or function. Thus, someone who wants to satisfy a fickle sweet tooth might be offered several varieties of chocolate and say, "Those are no good." The chocolate might be perfectly good—it just does not satisfy at the moment; it is of no good given present goals. Now, although "I have a bad ticker" and "those are no good" (uttered in the contexts cited) have much in common, they also seem different. Whether one has a bad heart does not seem to depend on the conscious goals of the individual, yet hearts do seem to be evaluated with respect to certain goals.

What determines the goals by which hearts are properly evaluated? This is a controversial matter. We want to say that hearts should be evaluated according to how well they perform their function. However, it is entirely unclear how to give a scientific explanation of a biological entity coming to have a function. We know how artifacts come to have functions: they are designed by entities that intend them to do things. Thus, a blender can have the functions of mixing, blending, whipping, and liquefying. And it is easy to determine that these are its functions—we look at the instructions or telephone the manufacturer. The functions of the blender are derived from, are dependent on, the intention of its designer. Of course, we may use the blender for some purpose of our own. We might use it as a paperweight or a vase. But this does not change its function.

Hearts are different. They do not come with instructions. We might suppose that they, like blenders, have a designer, but on most readings that supposition fails to ensure access to the designer's intentions. Furthermore, we were hoping for a scientific answer, one making reference only to natural phenomena, not supernatural ones. Some suppose that a marvelous accident has resulted in the existence of hearts, but that does nothing to help us understand why we are comfortable thinking that things such as hearts have functions in a way analogous to the way that blenders have functions.

Another approach to functions is Aristotelian. Stated roughly, the thesis is that everything has a natural function by virtue of the type of thing it is, and that the types of things are a matter of brute fact about the world. For Aristotle, natural objects were like seeds, waiting for the opportunity to express the nature inside, just as the acorn may wait through the winter to germinate and begin striving to grow into a mighty oak tree. In this picture, each natural object comes equipped with a *telos*, a goal or function, fulfilling which is the "good" for that thing.

The Aristotelian approach is very attractive, but has pained philosophers on several accounts. One is the metaphysical status of the "nature" that determines the *telos* of each object. In his *Physics*, Aristotle wrote, "...*nature is a source or cause of being moved and of being at rest in that to which it belongs primarily*..." (Aristotle 1941, 236). Later ancient and medieval philosophers developing this theme emphasized natures inhering in objects to such an extent that they were thought by some early modern philosophers to have been pantheistic, believing that little gods inhabited each thing.[5] Another difficulty is the Aristotelian tendency to see the fulfillment of the functions of natural objects as intrinsically good. This is particularly apparent in natural law theories in ethics, but plays an even broader role in Aristotle's system. The increasing sense in modern times that values cannot be universal, combined with the related but independent sense that the natural world is made up of observable facts, leads philosophers and scientists alike to reject the Aristotelian view despite its obvious advantages for projects such as ours.[6]

Non-Aristotelian accounts of natural function fall into historical (etiological) and nonhistorical categories. Historical accounts tell us that the causal history of an entity can make it so that the entity has a natural function. Consider, for instance, Ruth Millikan's account of proper function. This etiological theory portrays natural selection as responsible for determining proper function. The proper function of a biological organ or system is whatever ancestors of that organ or system did that contributed to the species surviving or proliferating (Millikan 1984, 316):

Underlining: that an organ or system has certain proper functions is determined by its *history*. It is *not* determined by its present properties, present structure, actual dispositions or actual functions.

Another approach relies on the current structure ("design" in a looser sense) of the object without reference to the history of the object. Robert Cummins (1993), for instance, maintained that we can come to conclusions about the functions of biological entities such as organs or systems of organs by analyzing their current capacities and those of their parts. Morphologist M. J. S. Rudwick (1998) held that functions can be discovered through examination of current structures of biological systems, a sort of reverse reverse-engineering.

Larry Wright (1998) emphasized the explanatory role of function ascriptions: ". . . when we say the heart beats in order to pump blood, we are ordinarily taken to be offering an explanation of why the heart beats" (65). His analysis of function ascriptions is as follows:

The function of X is Z means . . .
(a) X is there because it does Z,
(b) Z is a consequence (or result) of X's being there

The sense of "because" in (a) is explanatory; it is not there to cite the causal history that led to the presence of X, but to help us understand what X is doing there now.

Thus we have several different ways of accounting for our intuition that some biological entities such as hearts have functions. (I will not choose among them.) What they have in common is that they set up criteria for evaluation. Hearts are designed to pump blood; they exist to pump blood; it is their nature to pump blood; they are reproduced because of their blood-pumping capacity. All of these statements allow us to evaluate hearts. If a heart is designed to pump blood, then one that fails to do this well (assuming it is in the appropriate environment) is a bad specimen of its kind. (Of course, it could also be the case that the design is poor.) If a heart has been reproduced *because of* its blood-pumping capacity, one that fails to do this well is either a bad heart or the result of a poor mechanism of selection.

I want to emphasize here that the attribution of functions to objects underwrites evaluations, even for natural objects. Indeed, I suggest that what we mean when we use certain biological terms such as "heart" or "kidney" may be approximated as follows: a thing that is supposed to perform a function ϕ and hence can be evaluated according to how well it succeeds in performing ϕ under normal circumstances. The truth of this suggestion would not let the metaphysician off the hook of having to give some explanation of how there could be such a thing in the world as to fit this meaning. However, it can tell us a great deal both about what biological scientists are up to and about what has motivated so many philosophers to search for an adequate theory of natural function. Even if philosophers cannot find an adequate theory of natural function, this does not change the fact that biological scientists (including medical researchers) apply function terms to organs and systems in ways that structure evaluations of these organs and systems.

The notion of goal-directedness is important to understanding what it is to have a function in the sense that interests us here. Not everything that is said to have a function is itself goal directed, however. The function of a clock's pendulum is to regulate the mechanism, although it is really *our* goal that the pendulum regulate the mechanism, not the goal of the pendulum itself. Biological entities with intrinsic natural functions are a different matter. Although they may not adopt conscious goals, they are still said to aim at achievements that are independent of outside interests.

Ernest Nagel (1998) suggested that many philosophers fail to recognize important differences between function and goal-directedness. Goal ascriptions ". . . state some outcome or goal toward which certain activities of an organism or its parts are directed." Goal ascriptions he contrasted with "function ascriptions." Function ascriptions, he says, identify the actual effects or activities of some entity. Nagel admitted that "[s]ome biologists use the words 'goal' and 'function' interchangeably . . . possibly because the distinctions are not relevant to the tasks on which they are engaged" (199).

Nagel is right to point out, among other things, that goal ascriptions imply intentionality in the goal-directed entity much more strongly than do function ascriptions. However, in emphasizing the effects of functional entities, his theory is inadequate in accounting for entities that have a function that they are unable to perform.

Goal-directedness—aiming at something—is important to understanding biological function, because what fails to perform its function fails to reach a goal. Depending on what theory of biological function we adopt, we might think it impossible for biological entity E to have the function of ϕ-ing unless some, or even many, Es have succeeded in ϕ-ing in the past. However, it is certainly possible that a particular E has the function of ϕ-ing even if it has never succeeded at ϕ-ing. Obviously, a heart does not aim at a goal in the same way that I do. However, we evaluate it as if it did.

The Unity of Science and the New Biology

Biologists and medical scientists faced with the philosopher's tale tend to be indignant and bemused. They tend to be bemused by the fuss philosophers make over functions and goal-directedness. These they find obvious and relatively unproblematic. They are indignant in the face of the picture of the special sciences portrayed in A Philosophical Tale I.[7] Surely philosophers have noticed that biological sciences no longer have their own set of terms, terms wholly distinct from those of physics and chemistry! Modern genetics and pharmaceutical research, to name just two areas, make extensive use of chemical terms and types, just as orthopedics makes use of physics.

Biological scientists also take issue with the claim that their science is one of exception-prone principles. Once we allow them the use of physics and chemistry, explanations of failure of function come clearly into view. For instance, we can explain disruption of neural transmission, a biological function, by citing the presence of plaque, by noting a physical tangle in the neural structure, or by identifying a mutation or trauma.

All of this suggests that science is unified much more strongly than Fodor's picture of the special sciences would suggest. When scientists are entitled to whatever terms they need to solve problems that interest them, disciplinary distinctions become more an indication of the administrative structure of the university than of anything else. Indeed, with some prompting (a chemist of my acquaintance would admit that he accepts this view only after I promised not to tell his undergraduates), one can get some scientists to say that there are no really distinct scientific disciplines and that, instead, there is *just science*.

There is still something to say about the character of medical science even if medical science is simply part of a broader enterprise called science. The explanatory options regarding disrupted neural transmission are far simpler than our understanding of what causes most diseases. The epidemiologist's explanations commonly cite a number of factors, tendencies, and probabilities. Paul Thagard (2000) identified these as instances of what he called "causal network instantiation." "Causal network" refers to multiple interrelated factors. "Instantiation" occurs when we assign roles to some combination of these factors in an effort to explain the etiology of a particular patient's condition (Thagard 2000, 254). In this picture, explanation of disease is not deductive or statistical; neither does it cite a single cause. Instead, it "produces a kind of narrative explanation of why a person gets sick" (Thagard 2000, 271), which makes reference to the patient's relationship to some of the factors in the causal network (that commonly have only probabilistic causal connections to the disease explained). The causal network may cite factors using the language of physical, chemical, genetic, psychological, or environmental science.

However, even if there is just science and we are able to fill in ceteris paribus conditions of biological generalizations with physical and chemical explanations, normativity still plays a central role in biological (and perhaps some other) quadrants of science. Indeed, even Thomas Szasz (2000), a stalwart defender of the objective character of physical disease attributions, wrote, "Bodily diseases, conventionally defined, are undesirable [sic] deviations from objectively identifiable *biological norms*."[8] If the philosopher's tale helps bring philosophers to accept the legitimacy in science of the kind of normativity I have been describing, perhaps it was worth annoying the scientists a bit.

Normativity and Concepts of Health

Our philosophical tale was intended to show that talk of functions and goal-directed activity is a legitimate part of legitimate science. The significance of this is that we need not be prejudiced against normative theories of health, even if we are looking for a theory that can be part of science proper.

Four positions are available with respect to the role that normativity plays in health. First, some theories suggest that certain states are healthy and hence intrinsically valuable. They identify certain states as healthy and hold that the status of these states as healthy makes them desirable (good, ideal, or valuable) in themselves, and not just because they are useful as a means to another valued end. For such theories, certain conditions have intrinsic value, value that is not dependent on a particular community or individual.

According to these intrinsic normativity theories, the value that healthy states have is different from the value certain states may have due to contingent, even accidental, facts of agreement among individuals. For instance, we could imagine a world at which having long hair is universally valued because it is part of the socially constructed aesthetic of every society at that world. At such a world, having long hair would have value, not intrinsically, but because of societal agreement, which is extrinsic to hair length. This contrasts with the value attributed to healthy states by intrinsic normativity theories. One example of a state often believed to hold intrinsic value is the state of being alive. Many people believe that human life is valuable in itself, that being alive is always better than the alternative. They believe that human life has value even if no one recognizes that it does. Another familiar view that attributes intrinsic normativity to certain states is the Aristotelian view that such a thing as "the good" exists for human beings.[9]

A second type of theory posits that healthy states do not have intrinsic normativity, but are nonnormative. According to these nonnormativist theories, whether a system is healthy is neither good nor bad. In this view, people may value health for any number of reasons, but the value is independent of what states are healthy. That is, a value that health has is merely the result of people wanting to be in healthy states in order to get something else. In such a view, the value of health is like the value of gold. Gold is not intrinsically valuable; we want more gold only because of the things we can buy when we have it, and in many situations it would not be valued at all. However, whether it is valued does not affect whether it is in fact gold. Whether a given metal nugget is gold is a matter of chemical fact that by itself carries no evaluative force. Similarly, the nonnormativist wants to say that whether a given state is healthy is a matter of biomedical fact that by itself carries no evaluative force. Nonnormativist theories claim scientific objectivity.

Relativist theories, the third type, propose that whether a state is healthy depends entirely on whether it is considered healthy by the relevant individual or group, and not on anything intrinsic to the state itself. These theories involve what we might call *extrinsic normativity*. (It is conceivable that the extrinsic determination of health would be value free. A theory that proposed this would be nonnormativist. We will not consider such theories here, and reserve the term "relativism" for normativist theories.) In relativist theories, an extrinsic determination is entirely responsible for whether the state is healthy.

Note how relativism about health differs from nonnormativist and intrinsic normativist theories. Our example of the world in which long hair is a universal but socially determined value is useful for exploring what a relativist might say. Suppose that having long hair is considered healthy in all communities at this world. The relativist might say that what makes having long hair healthy at this world are the contingent values of the communities, that any community might have had different values, and hence having long hair *would not be healthy* in communities (at other worlds or at ours) that did not value it in this way. Following the conventions of ethics, we may call those theories *relativist* that hold that relevant values are those of an entire community, and *subjectivist* that hold that relevant values are those of the individual.

However, even if what counts as health depends on what individuals or communities contingently value, that does not mean that the definition of health has to advocate some values over others or accept a view in which health is valuable only instrumentally or extrinsically, if at all. I want to propose a theory of a fourth kind, a theory of health that characterizes certain states as being valuable neither intrinsically nor merely because they are useful, but rather because of their being in an appropriate relationship to an individual's actual values. By building variability into the theory in this way, such a view can accommodate variations in human goals that are recognized by the relativist and also take into account the important intuition that health is intrinsically good. Such a view might claim that certain states are healthy not in themselves but because they allow an individual to reach actual goals. We do not say that *a healthy state is valuable* because it allows us to reach or strive for goals, but rather that *a state is healthy* because it allows us to reach or strive for our goals. For want of a better term, I call this approach *embedded instrumentalism*.

Chapter 2 explores embedded instrumentalism in detail and defends a particular theory of health. In preparation, it is prudent to examine other theories of health so that we may become familiar with the territory.

Boorse on Disease and Illness

Christopher Boorse's (1977) biostatistical theory of health is the most widely discussed theory in the literature. In broad strokes, it states that health is statistically normal biological functioning. That is, a system is healthy if it is performing its biological functions well enough to count as typical for what Boorse calls its "reference class."

Boorse's full account goes as follows (1977, 555, 567):

1. The *reference class* is a natural class of organisms of uniform functional design; specifically, an age group of a sex of a species.

2. A *normal function* of a part or process within members of the reference class is a statistically typical contribution by it to their individual survival and reproduction.

3. A *disease* is a type of internal state which is either an impairment of normal functional ability, i.e., a reduction of one or more functional abilities below typical efficiency, or a limitation on functional ability caused by environmental agents.

4. *Health* is the absence of disease.

The reference class is a set of actual organisms. They must be of the same gender as the organism whose health is being evaluated because different genders have different sets of biological functions; they must be of the same age group because certain functions (e.g., growth) are different at different ages, and also because this allows us to avoid applying the term 'disease' to normal changes due to aging.

Having identified the (nonnormative) statistical normality concept of health as the one applied in medical theory, Boorse suggested that the concept of health applied in medical practice is related but different. It is set in contrast to illness rather than disease, where ". . . illnesses are merely a subclass of diseases, namely, those diseases that have certain normative features reflected in the institutions of medical practice" (1975, 56). Those diseases not treated in medical practice as bad are not illnesses.

Boorse is not the only one who embraced a distinction between disease and illness, with emphasis on the distinctively normative character of illness. Helman (1981) accepted the distinction as is. He and Mordacci and Sobel (1998) distinguished between disease and illness in a different but somewhat parallel way; Fulford (1989) maintained that diseases form a subset of illness rather than vice versa. Another approach, taken by Culver and Gert (1982), proposed that the concept of a malady is the most promising for explicating the normative aspect of health-related concepts.

Boorse's analysis of the theoretical concept of health (opposed to disease) is nonnormative. No values are involved in one's place in the distribution of biological measures. Like its theoretical counterpart, Boorse's clinical notion of health (opposed to illness) also does not attribute intrinsic value to healthy states. As it tells us that whether a state is unhealthy depends on (extrinsic) negative valuation in the practices of the medical community, it is a form of relativism. A remarkable feature of the theory is the claim that no condition can be an illness that is not also a disease.

Boorse's biostatistical theory is attractive. It seems to allow for an objective, scientific view of medicine and explains both the normativity and variability of diagnosis and treatment. Several compelling objections have been raised against it, however. Lennert Nordenfelt (1993a, 279) highlighted four. First, it is not adequately prepared to deal with the truly "great variation of normal values. . . ." Second, it does not consider how some organisms can maintain health by compensating for a lack of function in some area: "a subnormal value of a particular function can be compensated for by a supernormal value of a neighbouring function with the same net result." Third, the biostatistical theory does not allow for environmental factors affecting an entire population. (This objection was addressed in Boorse 1975.) Fourth, Boorse uses normative language in describing and developing his putatively nonnormative account of health.

Whereas others commenting on Boorse's theory have taken issue with the absence (or presence) of normativity (cf. Engelhardt 1996, chapter 5) and the emphasis on systems and mechanisms rather than on whole persons,[10] I want to draw attention to Boorse's concept of a "reference class." My concern is not with the general idea that health might be some relation to a comparison class. Rather, it is with the role of a comparison class of actually existing organisms. Consider the following passage:

... the subject matter of comparative physiology is a series of ideal types of organisms: the frog, the hydra, the earthworm, the starfish, the crocodile, the shark, the rhesus monkey, and so on. The idealization is of course statistical, not moral or esthetic or normative in any other way. (Boorse 1977, 557)

While admitting that there may be no disease-free crocodile, Boorse suggested that the distribution of levels of functioning among systems in the actual crocodile population is such that the composite idea of a croc with average levels of functioning for each of its systems will allow us to draw conclusions about what constitutes a normal crocodile.

This theory is meant to invoke species design. In fact, Boorse writes that "Our interest in species design is that we wish to analyze health as conformity to it" (Boorse 1977, 558). Boorse did not see that taking statistical normality to indicate species design is an illicit inference from a fact to a value. This is presumably because he did not see species design as determining a value. However, species design is not value neutral. It indicates how something is supposed to be; it involves normativity. We may not mind when certain things deviate from how they were supposed to be, but this does not take away from the fact that they were supposed to be a certain other way. But if we want to talk about species design, we are immediately introducing the possibility, even the likelihood, that members of the reference classes identified by Boorse may deviate from the ideal in such a way that their internal states are *all, for every member of the class*, impaired.

The nonnormative statistical variety of normality yields a specimen that is ideal in the sense of being a composite rather than an actual member of the reference class. But we should not confuse this sort of ideal with the normative sort. Even if Boorse did not confuse these two senses of ideal, he did seem to confuse the epistemological and the metaphysical. I say this because his theory makes more sense if we think of the reference class as *evidence for claims about normality*, than if we think of it as being *that on which normality supervenes*. Constructing a concept of an ideal crocodile based on an examination of statistically typical states of a reference class of crocodiles may be the best way to generate justified beliefs about the species design of crocodiles. And this may be so even if, as I suggest, being the statistically typical croc and being a croc with systems that perform as designed are quite different concepts. We only hope (for the crocodiles' sake at least) that they coincide in the actual population.

Given that these two ideals may not come together in the actual case, we might imagine how we might respond if they in fact did not. For instance, perhaps 60 percent of the reference class has gastric ulcers, which impair digestive function. We can specify that these ulcers are not the kind enabled by infection, so they do not count as caused by an environmental agent. In this case we would reject the usual reference class as inappropriate for helping us to determine the ideal specimen and look to some other reference. So it seems that the ideal relevant to our judgments about health should not be the reference class of actual organisms (as Boorse would have it), but rather that our judgment about what constitutes the appropriate reference class is determined by the ideal. And yet it is unclear how we are to determine the ideal without some reference to actual organisms.

Boorse thought that he avoided objections such as mine, generally the problem of universal diseases (he did not claim to have solved the problem of universal genetic diseases), by distinguishing in part 3 of his definition between internal states and external agents (Boorse 1977, 566–67). However, there is no principled way to distinguish between internal and external. Are viruses internal or external? What about bacteria such as *Escherischia coli* that exist in normal symbiosis with humans in certain parts of our bodies but are unhealthy when present in other parts? Consider mitochondria, which are thought to have arisen from intracellular parasites that have become symbiotic with us. Problems with mitochondria are responsible for macular degeneration—is this an external or internal condition? In addition, internal states would include problems with expression of genes even when the genes themselves are normal. Such congenital defects are not genetic diseases. So it seems that universal genetic diseases are not the only conditions that cause difficulty for Boorse's definition.

Fulford's "Reverse View"

In *Moral Theory and Medical Practice* (1989), Fulford defended what he called a reverse view of disease and illness. One of his main concerns was mental illness. He acknowledged the dominance of views, such as those of Boorse and Szasz, according to which the legitimacy of mental illness rests on the degree to which it is analogous to the presumably more objective and scientific notions of physical illness and disease. As we have seen, Szasz, Boorse, and others who wanted to eschew relativism by holding tight to science took dysfunction and (physical) disease to be the central and most logically basic concepts in medicine.

Against these views, Fulford contended that illness is in fact the more central concept:

. . . for patients, at least, the logical priority of 'illness' . . . corresponds with the actual *experience* of illness; for the complaint normally precedes the diagnosis of the complaint; knowledge *that* something is wrong normally precedes the question *what* is wrong, let alone questions about possible *causes* of what is wrong. (70)

In ordinary usage, Fulford noted, disease terms "would be used typically . . . to say *what* is wrong with someone who is ill" (63). This reverse view of the relationship between disease and illness does accord with a common sort of clinical experience: one feels ill and reports to the doctor to find out what is wrong. The frequent repetition of this course of events lends credence to the reverse view. Of course, the person may be wrong about whether he is ill. For example, he might mistake a benign mole for a cancerous one.

Another sort of clinical experience, raises questions for the reverse view. In some cases an individual goes to the doctor because of a condition that the physician agrees is statistically abnormal (and thus a disease in Boorse's account) but does not require treatment. Consider, for example, a young person in late adolescence who is experiencing a late growing episode, or a twelve-year-old who is growing at a rate that is slower than normal. Such a youngster could leave the clinic believing that he was somewhat unusual but not ill or diseased. Fulford's reverse view, although insightful, may not characterize all medical encounters quite accurately.

Another important aspect of Fulford's theory is his understanding of illness in terms of *failure of ordinary action*: ". . . failure of . . . 'ordinary' doing in the apparent absence of obstruction and/or opposition" (109). This failure can include the simple inability to do something (such as move one's arm) or failure of one's beliefs and desires to work together into a coherent set of reasons for action that allow one to navigate the world (as in the case of schizophrenia and certain other psychological illnesses; see Fulford 1989, chapter 8). The emphasis on *ordinary* doing allows Fulford to distinguish between illness and disability, where disability is a state affecting what one can ordinarily do (see Fulford 1989, 125).

This theory has several features that should be highlighted. In identifying illness (the notion that something is *wrong*) as the most basic concept in medicine, his account is normative. Emphasis on the role of action accounts for three other important features. First, it draws attention to the patient as a conscious, whole person rather than just a body with systems that may or may not be functioning to species-typical levels. Second, the emphasis on action builds in a wide range of variability in states that will count as unhealthy due to the wide range of things that people "ordinarily" do. We see, also, that Fulford's theory links health to goal-directed activity. Ordinary action involves trying (and succeeding) to do something that one at least minimally wants to do.

Conclusion

This chapter defended the legitimacy of teleological terms such as "function" and "goal-directed" in medical science and related them to the concept of normativity. Our four-fold taxonomy of the roles that normativity can play in a theory of health helped shape our exploration of Christopher Boorse's influential biostatistical theory and K. W. M. Fulford's reverse view. Normativity, goal-directedness, and biological variation arose as central to biological science and hence to theories of health. These concepts will play important roles in the theories discussed and defended in the next chapter and, indeed, the rest of this book.

2

A Proposal: Embedded Instrumentalism

The first chapter identified four types of theories of health that differ in the role played by values (normativity). First are nonnormative theories, according to which whether a state of a person or organism is healthy is just a matter of fact; they say nothing about what is good or bad, or even about what is valued or disvalued. Second are theories that hold that being healthy is inherently valuable, so that when we say that a state is healthy we are pointing out something good about that state. That is, the goodness of healthy states is intrinsic to the states and independent of judgment about them. The third set of theories attributes extrinsic value to healthy states. Saying that a state is healthy draws attention not to some goodness inherent in the state itself, but rather to the fact that the speaker (or the community) values that state in a certain way.

In this chapter we will consider the type of theory I call embedded instrumentalism. I do not mean theories according to which there is such a state as health and that state is valuable only as a means to something else. Instead, I mean theories according to which health is something like *whatever state allows the person to reach or strive for his or her goals*, where the goals are actual goals of an individual, and are not assumed to have value except insofar as the person in fact values them.[1] Embedded instrumentalist theories can be understood as holistic in the sense that they "take the human being as a whole into account" (Nordenfelt 1993b, 321).

I hold that it is, ceteris paribus, better for people to be in a state that allows them to reach or strive for their goals than for them to be in a state in which that is not possible. Because this is the case without the individual having to have a further, second-order goal of being able to fulfill his or her goals, embedded instrumentalist theories of health are normativist. However, they differ from intrinsic normativism in claiming that physical or psychological states are not healthy in themselves but only insofar as they stand in the right relationship to the goals (and perhaps other conditions) of the person whose states they are. They differ from extrinsic normativity theories such as relativism in that embedded instrumentalist theories identify one concept of health as the correct one.

I maintain that the appropriate analysis of health is an embedded instrumentalist theory. First, I will explain this approach by claiming that it can be understood as an analogue to the instrumental rationality concepts of epistemology defended by Larry Laudan and Richard Foley, among others. Recognizing that the goals of an individual considered from the point of view of biology and the goals of the individual considered as an agent in the world might be different, I introduce a distinction between *the health of an individual qua organism* and *the health of an individual qua person*. I then propose that this distinction characterizes evaluations made by patients and health care professionals better than the widely discussed distinction between disease and illness.

A Philosophical Analogy—Instrumental Rationality

I understand the embedded instrumentalist concept of health to be the analogue in philosophy of medicine of the instrumental rationality concept of justification in efforts to naturalize epistemology and the philosophy of science. For instance, although in his essay "Epistemology Naturalized" Quine (1986) held that normative epistemology is no longer a viable enterprise, later he identified certain goals as important to scientists (and others) as they decide what theories to accept as true. These values, including simplicity, consistency, and truth, have no intrinsic value. They are, however, the things we aim for when we are doing science. Epistemology then becomes "... a branch of engineering. It is the technology of truth seeking, or, in more cautiously epistemic terms, prediction" (Quine 1986, 663). Epistemology in this picture is about identifying the means to a particular end: truth.

Larry Laudan noted that the aims of science (and hence of epistemology) are subject to change. "Central to my reading of the epistemic enterprize, although not crucial to naturalistic epistemology per se, is the idea that the aims of science in particular and of inquiry in general have exhibited certain significant shifts through time" (Laudan 1990, 48). Whereas scientists might always be willing to say that their goal is knowledge, our ideas of what counts as scientific knowledge have certainly varied. Aristotle's scientific *episteme* had as its object unchanging essences, and was the result of demonstration in the sense of deductive syllogisms.[2] Today scientific knowledge is oriented to quantitative data, is subject to refutation from contrary data, avoids talk of essences, and often even avoids talk of causes (Laudan 1990, 49). Science may always have knowledge as its goal, but if what constitutes knowledge can be different in different situations or environments, what we are aiming at has its value extrinsically and not intrinsically. Rational scientific practice then becomes not those practices aimed at some particular goal, but rather practices aimed at whichever goals are contingently determined to be scientific by a given community at a given time.

R. N. Giere (1989) distinguished between "categorical" or "unconditional" rationality, which would be based on objective, independent standards of justification, and "conditional" or "instrumental" rationality:

> To be instrumentally rational is simply to employ means believed to be conducive to achieving desired goals. . . . [T]here is also a more *objective* sense of instrumental rationality which consists in employing means that are not only believed to be, but are *in fact* conducive to achieving desired goals. (Giere 1989, 379–80, quoted in Siegel 1996, S117)

According to the theory of instrumental rationality, engaging in the sort of activities that help us to reach our goals for revising our theory of the world is *constitutive* of rationality. In a view such as Giere's, being rational (or thinking scientifically) is not a matter of applying some universal, unchanging method to reach universal, unchanging goals. Rather, it is about applying effective methods to reach contingent, possibly changing goals.

The fact that the goals are contingent and may change does not mean that applying appropriate methods to reach them is not what it means to be rational. Note that we are working with one concept of rationality that allows for variability. It is not relativistic, yet it is context sensitive and it allows for objective evaluation of whether a particular inference is rational or irrational.

I want to say that being in a state that allows us to reach a certain set of goals is constitutive of health, that to be in such a state is what it is to be healthy. Such a theory of health, like its analogue in epistemology, is not relativistic. It is context sensitive and yet allows for objective evaluation of whether a particular state is healthy or unhealthy.

Pörn, Whitbeck, Nordenfelt, and Seedhouse

Ingmar Pörn's equilibrium model of health offers an embedded instrumentalist account.

Health is the state of a person which obtains exactly when his repertoire [of abilities] is adequate relative to his profile of goals. (Pörn 1984, 5)

In this view, health is a match, or equilibrium between one's goals and one's abilities. Thus someone who is ill can become healthy either by adjusting goals or by adjusting abilities.

Pörn (1993) introduced a third factor into the equilibrium: the environment in which the individual seeks to meet his or her goals. In this enriched version of the equilibrium theory of health:

If the agent is deficient in adaptedness the deficiency must be described in terms of an inadequate repertoire [of abilities], an inappropriate environment or an unrealistic goal profile, or in terms of some combination of these. (Pörn 1993, 300)

Pörn distinguished between time-specific adaptedness and generalized adaptedness. He also offered a discussion of the ranking of personal goals, to which we will return later.

Pörn's position provides a helpful way of describing many cases. Consider the athlete who desperately wants to be able to run a two-minute mile, but can only run a six-minute mile. This can be described as a state of disequilibrium in which the individual's goals are set too high relative to the individual's abilities. Another example might be the man who aspires to be a fashion model but does not have the appropriate bone structure. In such cases it makes sense to recommend treatment that would adjust the patient's profile of goals. However, with other problems such as hypertension or melanoma, adjusting goals to accommodate the condition would not be a way to make a patient healthy.

Caroline Whitbeck (1981b) offered another embedded instrumentalist theory in which health is an individual's "psychophysiological capacity" to behave in ways that are "supportive of the person's goals, projects, and aspirations in a wide variety of situations" (620). Like Pörn's, this account of health has the virtue of simplicity. Perhaps the key difference between the theories lies in their respective uses of 'adequate' and 'appropriate'. Appropriate responses *aim at* a goal; adequate responses *satisfy* a goal. As Nordenfelt pointed out (1995, 66), it is easier to respond appropriately than it is to respond adequately. This makes Whitbeck's theory weaker than Pörn's—Whitbeck will count more individuals among the healthy than will Pörn. Whitbeck's theory is also more akin to the one I am defending in that responding in a way that is supportive of one's goals is much like striving to satisfy one's goals. More on this below.

Nordenfelt's embedded instrumentalist theory emphasizes the centrality of what he called the "vital goals" of the individual. The following is his definition of health:

P is completely healthy, if and only if P has the ability, given standard circumstances, to realise all his or her vital goals. (Nordenfelt 1993a, 280)

That is, P is *unhealthy* (ill) if and only if P is unable to realize some or all of his vital goals in standard circumstances. This theory allows for degrees of health and illness.

Nordenfelt (1995) defined the vital goals of the individual as those "necessary and together sufficient for [the individual's] minimal happiness" (90). What counts as a vital goal is determined in part by the individual and in part by environmental factors. These relevant factors include the physical environment, the cultural environment, and the degree to which resources are available to the individual given these factors.

Since the cultural environment is important in Nordenfelt's theory, questions about health may be answered differently in different societies. However, this variability does not mean that his theory is a variety of relativism:

. . . a man in good health in [society] S_1 may have properties quite different from a man in good health in S_2.

Observe, however, that strictly speaking this does not mean that the two societies have different *concepts* of health. . . . The *concept* is the same, but since what counts as standard societal circumstances differs in S_1 and S_2 the reference class of healthy people will differ in nature for the two. (Nordenfelt 1995, 120)

Like Pörn, Nordenfelt made clear how embedded instrumentalism allows for the variability we find in judgments about health while capturing what these judgments have in common. However, I believe that in emphasizing "standard societal circumstances," Nordenfelt left inadequate room for the role that the preferences of individuals play in medical decisions. We will discuss Nordenfelt further in our consideration of goals later in this chapter.

Yet another embedded instrumentalist definition of health is offered by David Seedhouse, who described the "optimum state of health" for a person as a "set of conditions which fulfil or enable a person to work to fulfil his or her realistic chosen and biological potentials" (1986, 61). Some conditions will be equally important to everyone and others will vary from individual to individual (Seedhouse 1986, 61). Like Nordenfelt, Seedhouse worked into his theory both the universal and the variable. The universal is captured by the inclusion of "biological potentials."

Matthew Clayton (1999) raised an important worry about embedded instrumentalist theories in a review of Nordenfelt's book *Talking about Health: A Philosophical Dialogue*. It is worth quoting at length:

The worry is that some who have few ambitions in life and are, therefore, content with less by way of physical or mental functioning will be regarded as less urgent medical cases than others, even when their modest ambitions are an effect of their low level of functioning in the first place. . . . Many would regard it as counterintuitive to prioritise the interests of those whose need for medical treatment is a consequence of their adoption of a lifestyle which is more demanding from the point of view of the mental and physical resources required to pursue it.

Clayton's worry drives at the core of embedded instrumentalism. Embedded instrumentalist theories seek to find the balance between two demands put on theories of health: standards of health have to be flexible to allow for different circumstances and goals, but they also must capture our intuition that health really does not vary greatly from individual to individual. These two demands lead to conflicts in our intuitions about what is healthy in particular situations.[3]

I believe we can address these demands and build on the groundwork laid by Pörn and Nordenfelt by coupling an embedded instrumentalist theory with a distinction between the health of an individual considered as a biological organism and the health of the same individual considered as a moral agent.

Health of Organisms and Health of Persons

Human beings have complex and overlapping sets of goals. In this section, I describe briefly the ways in which it makes sense to say that thinking of an individual as a biological organism involves attributing to that person a set of goals. (We discussed goal-directedness in chapter 1.) This way of thinking offers one set of answers about what healthy states are for each individual. Next, I point out that there is often (and perhaps usually) less than comprehensive coincidence between the goals of an individual considered as a biological organism and the goals of that same individual as an agent in the world. Therefore, we can expect that the goals of the individual considered as an agent in the world will pick out a set of states as healthy for the individual that may be different from the states picked out with reference to biological goals. What it is for the individual qua organism to be healthy will often not be the same as what it is for that same individual qua person to be healthy. This way of developing the embedded instrumentalist approach to health arose in collaboration with Andrew E. Budson. (Richman and Budson 2000a, b). I therefore refer to the theory defended here as the Richman–Budson theory of health.

Even in their doings that are disconnected from actual beliefs and desires, organisms exhibit activity that can be described as goal directed. We are able to explain many of the things that occur in organisms with reference to some desired future state. Why does the body produce an unusually large number of white blood cells? To be rid of a current infection. Why does the heart beat? To circulate blood.

As discussed in chapter 1, serious problems with such explanations arise if we take them to have metaphysical implications. Hearts simply cannot have intentions and goals in the core sense. Even if we want to couch our attribution of goals to organisms (considered as biological entities) in terms of functions, problems still exist. Our primary model for understanding what it is to have a function invokes the notion of a design plan and hence a designer. A blender, to take our old example, has the function it does because some designer intended it to do certain things. I want to remain neutral with respect to whether the human organism has a designer. The most promising theories of function that avoid implying the existence of a designer explain functions in terms of (past) causes rather than goals for the future, raising doubts about whether they are truly teleological.

Nevertheless, functional explanations remain useful and intuitive in the biological sciences and are standard in medicine. We identify many occurrences in the body as aimed at achieving a goal and doing a better or worse job of it. We can usually agree on what the goals of these occurrences are. Although metaphysicists may not have a place in their pictures of the world for the "goal" of the renal system, biologists and physicians do.

No proof is necessary for the claim that individuals considered as persons, as moral agents in the world, have goals. These may be unclear, hidden or vague, but they will be identifiable, at least in broad outline. Although the goals of individuals understood as biological organisms are mostly the same, the goals of individuals as moral agents differ from person to person.

Three brief examples will illustrate our distinction between health of organisms and health of persons.

1. A person with untreated bipolar disease may find a hypomanic state helpful for a personal goal of finishing a project or finding creative inspiration. On the other hand, untreated bipolar disease is definitely unhealthy for the organism, frequently causing promiscuity leading to disease, the spending of large sums of money leading to huge debt, and so on.[4]

2. Many question why such a huge number of cases of attention deficit–hyperactivity disorder (ADHD) is diagnosed—about 4 percent of school-age children (Holden 1999)—when previously it (and its nominal

predecessor, minimal brain dysfunction) was relatively uncommon. One explanation may be that the goals of persons in our society have changed from survival to schooling. Mild ADHD may actually be productive and healthy for an individual qua organism in environments where hypervigilance and quick reflexes are required to survive. However, even mild cases may cause disruption of attention sufficient to be unhealthy for the same individual qua person if the goal of the person is to perform well in school.

3. Ovulatory menstrual cycles may be completely healthy in a woman qua organism, since one of the goals of organisms is to reproduce. However, if a woman's personal goals require that she avoid pregnancy, this state may be thought of as unhealthy for the woman qua person and treated with medication to cause anovulatory cycles.

An additional example can illustrate an important feature of our theory: what constitutes health for an individual can change from one day to the next. Oliver Sacks (1970) gave the example in his book, *The Man Who Mistook His Wife for a Hat*, of Witty Ticcy Ray, a businessman from nine to five and drummer on weekends. Ray found Tourette syndrome disruptive to most aspects of his life, interfering with both personal and business relationships, although not with his drumming. Because disruption of personal relationships may lead to reduced chances of mating and reproducing, and disruption of business relationships may lead to difficulty obtaining food and shelter, Tourette syndrome was unhealthy for Ray qua organism. He wanted treatment with medication, which had the desired effect of restoring his personal and business relationships. However, the drug had the undesirable effect of impairing his drumming performance. Although drumming had no survival or reproductive value, it had personal value. Monday through Friday, when he did not wish to drum, drug therapy produced health for both Ray qua organism and Ray qua person. On weekends when he wanted to drum, he did not take the drug, producing health for Ray qua person but disease for Ray qua organism. Luckily for Ray, the half-life of the medication was brief enough to allow him to hold off taking the drug before gigs, and thereby in a given week he could accomplish both organismal and (changing) personal goals.

I claimed early in chapter 1 that an adequate theory of health should be such that if two people disagree on whether a given state is healthy, it will either tell us that at least one of them is incorrect or give an account of how they can both be correct. The theory that I am defending satisfies this condition. As we learned from the discussion above, some disagreements will arise concerning whether a given condition is healthy in which one side is simply incorrect because the condition in question is not conducive to the individual meeting his or her goals. However, in other instances both sides will be correct, and this will be explained by noting that the individual is being considered in different lights by the disputing parties.

In chapter 1 we examined Christopher Boorse's influential biostatistical theory of health, with its distinction between illness and disease. How does this distinction differ from the distinction between the health of an organism and the health of a person in how it assesses conditions of individuals? Table 2.1 compares Boorse's treatment with the Richman–Budson treatment.

Boorse's analysis calls for treatment to "correct" conditions that help individuals reach their personal goals, and does not recognize as unhealthy other conditions in which treatment is necessary for them to reach these goals. Boorse's distinction between disease and illness is an attempt to accommodate the variable aspect of medicine. The effort falls short for two reasons. First, it limits the discussion of what conditions ought to be treated by health care professionals to those identified by medical theory as diseases. Second, the variety of opinions concerning what conditions ought to be treated is limited to the number of communities with established "institutions of medical practice." However, the examples presented above show that we can (and do) give credibility to a much wider variety of opinions than that. In short, our embedded instrumentalist theory offers evaluations of health that suggest treatment decisions more in accord with our intuitions about the best use of medical resources.

Development and Clarification

I have suggested that individuals are healthy when they are in a state that enables them to reach or strive for their goals. This theory is a

Table 2.1
Comparison of two theories of health

Condition	Theory	Application
Untreated bipolar disorder	Richman–Budson	Hypomanic state may make the disorder healthy for person. Unhealthy for organism.
	Boorse	A disease. An illness (treated as undesirable by "the institutions of medical science").
Mild attention deficit–hyperactivity disorder	Richman–Budson	Typically unhealthy for person (particularly those in our society). May or may not be healthy for organism, depending on environment.
	Boorse	A disease (certain areas of the brain functioning below statistical norm). An illness.
Ovulatory menstrual cycles	Richman–Budson	Unhealthy for woman who wants to avoid pregnancy. Healthy for organism.
	Boorse	Not a disease, except among females in age groups for which menstruation itself is unusual. Not an illness.
Treatment of Tourette syndrome in Oliver Sacks's Witty Ticcy Ray—Monday through Friday	Richman–Budson	Healthy for person because improves interpersonal relationships. Healthy for organism because improves interpersonal relationships.
	Boorse	Healthy because Tourette's is a disease. Healthy because Tourette's is an illness.
Treatment of Tourette syndrome in Oliver Sacks's Witty Ticcy Ray—Weekends	Richman–Budson	Unhealthy for person because impairs drumming performance. Healthy for organism because improves interpersonal relationships.
	Boorse	Healthy because Tourette's is a disease. Healthy because Tourette's is an illness.

Reprinted from Richman and Budson 2000b with permission of the publisher.

species of instrumentalism because of the role played by contingent goals. I called it an embedded instrumentalist theory to emphasize that being healthy is not a matter of aiming for the right goals, but involves a match between abilities and goals. In this way, the theory captures the normative implications of 'health' while avoiding problematic relativism. I also proposed that an embedded instrumentalist theory cannot stand without a corollary distinction between the health of organisms and the health of persons. In table 2.1 the proposed theory is applied to evaluate five possible cases and found to offer defensible and intuitive judgments.

It is important to note that the present formulation of our theory of health and its corollary distinction between the health of individuals qua persons and the health of individuals qua organisms are limited in significant ways. First, although the theory has implications for medical ethics that are explored in later chapters, it is not itself an ethical theory. That is, it is not a theory of what goals people ought to have, and is not meant to be such. The significance of this point will become clearer as the discussion unfolds.

Because few people would be satisfied with a life in which all of their goals were reached, I have specified that health is the ability to reach *or strive for* our goals. I have left this aspect unanalyzed in order to concentrate on the broader issues. I offer some remarks on striving near the end of this chapter.

A Note on Realism and Supervenience
In characterizing my theory as a metaphysics of health, I invite the question of whether it is a form of *realism* about health. Metaphysicists, or, as may be appropriate here, metaphysicians, are concerned with what the world is made up of. In deference to general guidelines concerning how to choose among competing theories, metaphysicians are particularly concerned to find the simplest theory that does the job of explaining what we take to be facts about the world. I do claim that there are facts about health. Thus I advocate a sort of cognitivism about health ascriptions. I also hold that health supervenes on certain other features of the world. That is, one's health status does not change unless some

other facts change; specifically, unless there is a change in ability or goal. Supervenience is a type of dependence relation, so that we can say that facts about health depend on facts about these other things. Thus I am not committed to the claim that health facts are among the most basic facts about the world. Let me explain what I mean as follows. Consider what God might have to do to create a world precisely identical to the present one. In the view I offer, God would have to create all the facts about our abilities and goals, but would not have to perform an additional act of creation to replicate the facts about health. These would just fall into place once the other facts are taken care of.

Health is multiply realizable—there are lots of ways to be healthy. When we judge that a given state is healthy, we are making an assertion about the relationship between a set of goals and a set of abilities. Thus we can speak of health as a *relation* holding between sets of goals and sets of abilities. Although I will continue to speak of individuals, persons, and organisms being healthy or unhealthy, my analysis tells us that such statements are made true or false by facts about pairs of related sets—sets of goals and sets of abilities.

Problems with Goals: Nordenfelt's Worries

Our embedded instrumentalist theory suggests that health is indexed to goals. Once we open the door to the idea that individuals qua organisms have goals, this part of the theory falls into place as a function of biological science. Now our difficulties come from the goals of individuals qua persons. Nordenfelt (1995) considered two types of embedded instrumentalist theories: one according to which the relevant goals are defined by *need* (where it is understood that all needs have some biological basis) and what he called *subject goal theories*, which are along the lines of the Richman–Budson theory of health of persons. Nordenfelt understood his "welfare" theory of health as a development of the basic idea driving subject goal (SG) theories, a development that preserves their successes and avoids their problems. He identified four issues as prima facie problematic for SG theories. I will use them to structure the discussion as we begin to develop and defend the Richman–Budson theory. Nordenfelt's issues are:

(a) The case of unrealistic persons with too high ambitions
(b) The case of the person with extremely low ambitions
(c) The case of counterproductive goals
(d) The restricted applicability—the SG–notion is only a notion of adult human health. (1995, 71)

Nordenfelt distinguished among the goals a subject might actually intend to fulfill and the subject's mere wants, such as the want a sports fan might have of meeting a favorite athlete. He understood SG theories to be about the subject's "intended goals."

(a) A person with unrealistically high goals is unlikely to be able to realize these goals. Although one or two unrealistic goals may just be indicative of idealism or ambition rather than of ill health, the individual with many unrealistic goals would indeed be deemed unhealthy by SG theories. The goals that count in this assessment are intended ones, and not mere wants. Although identifying this case as a prima facie problem, Nordenfelt was in the end willing to concur with the assessment of SG theories when the subject's entire set of goals is considered:

A person who is not justified in believing that a particular state of affairs is attainable and still makes this state an intended goal of his, is unrealistic with respect to this goal. If such a lack of realism obtains with regard to most of his intended goals then he has, according to the SG-theory, a low degree of health. (Nordenfelt 1995, 74)

Depending on how one understands the terms "justified" and "attainable," this characterization may count far too many goals as unrealistic. In any case, some individuals have goals they are *justified* in believing to be *un*attainable. This is a better description of unrealistic goals.

Nordenfelt did not consider unrealistically high goals to be barriers to accepting SG theories. This is important, though, because it suggests that we have to say something about how many or which goals are such that failure to be able to reach them is unhealthy. It also raises the related issue of degrees of health.

Surely there are degrees of health. Inability to reach or strive for one or two goals, particularly those not held very dearly and not essential to our continuing to exist as living beings, may make us less healthy, but often will not make us unhealthy *tout court*. We can make perfect sense of claims that someone's health has "taken a turn for the worse." Determining which combinations of abilities count as more or less healthy than certain others will be an inexact exercise, even in cases where we are given a specified set of personal (or biological) goals. The clearest ranking of sets of abilities will follow from clarification of the person's goals and of their relative importance to the individual.

(b) The case of the person with extremely low ambitions seems to pose a greater challenge for SG theories than does the case of the person with unrealistically high goals. People with extremely low ambitions are not homogeneous, however. Some people have low ambitions because they are slothful or lazy, others because they are impaired cognitively or emotionally. Consider a hypothetical lazy person, Mr. Sloth. Mr. Sloth's goals are to lie around and watch television all day. Suppose that, by coincidence, he possesses very limited abilities, as well, abilities minimally sufficient for this very limited set of goals. We are stipulating, however, that he has set his goals at a low level only because of his lazy character and independent of beliefs about his low level of abilities. What can we say about this person? If he is actually unable to engage in the pursuit of a richer set of goals, Mr. Sloth is not healthy qua organism; his body surely needs more activity to reach the goals at which *it* aims even though he is able to satisfy his personal goals. However, Mr. Sloth's failure to set higher goals for himself (qua person) is more a matter of moral than of medical evaluation. Qua organism, Mr. Sloth is unhealthy; qua individual, Mr. Sloth is more properly called immoral.

Nordenfelt failed to distinguish the lazy person from individuals in "chronic comas" and those who adjust their goals downward to an extremely low level because they believe their situation to be one in which low ambitions represent all that they are likely to achieve (see Nordenfelt 1995, 75). He saw SG theories as offering counterintuitive judgments concerning all of these people. Take, for instance, an individual in a persistent vegetative state, or PVS. (I take it that this is what Nordenfelt meant by "chronic comas.") As Nordenfelt admitted, such individuals "do not seem to have any ambitions at all" (75). According to a simple SG theory, an individual in a PVS either has no health status at all because he has no goals, or is perfectly healthy because one requires no abilities to reach no goals, and no abilities is approximately what this person has.[5]

The Richman–Budson theory can deal with these cases much better than can simple SG theories. If people in persistent vegetative states have no goals, they are not strictly speaking moral agents. To be a moral agent, they would have to make choices and perform intentional actions; typically, actions for which they might be blamed or praised. They perform no such actions. As they are not moral agents, they do not have a status with respect to health qua persons. But this does not mean that they have no health status whatever. We may still evaluate them with respect to health qua organisms.

Of course, we do tend to think that a person's goals are relevant to what happens to the person's body and property even after the person ceases to be, strictly speaking, a bearer of goals. Such thinking is no challenge to the Richman–Budson theory if we recognize its basis in the fact that these individuals still play a functional role in families and communities. It is out of respect for the institution of personhood and to fulfill our own duties that we respect the "intentions" of someone who will never again have personal goals, not out of an obligation to the body that remains in the hospital bed.

Those who have adjusted their goals downward to an extremely low level due to beliefs about their situation are quite a different story. Some cases of depression fall into this category. According to the *Diagnostic and Statistical Manual*, fourth edition (*DSM IV–TR*), diagnosis of major depressive episode requires, among other things, meeting five of nine criteria. Consider criterion 7 (2000, 356):

feelings of worthlessness or excessive or inappropriate guilt (which may be delusional) nearly every day (not merely self-reproach or guilt about being sick).

An individual may meet this criterion by virtue of having a particular kind of delusion. Delusion is, in turn, defined as:

A false belief based on incorrect inference about external reality that is firmly sustained despite what almost everyone else believes and despite what constitutes incontrovertible and obvious proof or evidence to the contrary. . . . When a false belief involves a value judgment, it is regarded as a delusion only when the judgment is so extreme as to defy credibility. (*DSM IV–TR* 2000, 821)

Criterion 7 suggests that feelings can be delusional even though a delusion is a false belief.[6] This can perhaps be understood if we take the feeling of worthlessness to be equivalent to a belief that one is worthless. "Worthlessness" has moral overtones, but it also suggests an assessment that the person is unable to do very much or unable to perform actions that are valued. Thus whereas in some people depression involves *inability* to reach goals, in others it involves a *false assessment of ability* that can lead to setting goals too low. Presumably, no individual would be diagnosed with depression on the basis of a true belief that he has low abilities (is "worthless"). Therefore, appropriate therapy for a depressed person with low goals is likely to involve efforts to revise false beliefs.[7] (We will see parallels in the discussion of body dysmorphic disorder below.)

(c) Cases of counterproductive goals include the dieter who wants to lose weight but also wants to eat lots of sweets, and the wild one who wants to spend a late night drinking at a bar despite also wanting to perform well at work the next morning.[8] Counterproductive goals are problematic for SG theories if we want health to be attainable even in principle—one cannot reach inconsistent goals at the same time. Nordenfelt addressed this issue by identifying what he called vital goals. Getting plastered every night down the pub will not count as a vital goal for anyone.

The Richman–Budson theory does not embrace Nordenfelt's distinction between vital and nonvital goals because it straddles, and hence blurs, the distinction between health of organisms and health of persons. We must find another way of coming to terms with these cases. To do so, we must first note that health cannot be measured at a particular instant, but must be considered over a period of time. Someone who at the moment has no desires because she is asleep or temporarily knocked unconscious does not thereby cease to have personal goals. Similarly, a merely transient goal should not be assigned a very important role in determining the health of an individual.

Perhaps we can be helped by Pörn's idea of a life plan. A life plan is made up of "goals for comprehensive segments of one's life" (Pörn 1993, 299). The life plan is the set of overarching goals that "give structure" to an individual's personal goals. It certainly is possible that getting plastered every night down the pub is part of the life plan for some person. As with the lazy person, we might consider this individual to be immoral. However, it would not be surprising for such a person to present at a physician's office with the complaint that he can no longer "hold his liquor" the way he used to.

Could an individual's life plan be inconsistent? Certainly. And the individual might persist in holding onto the life plan even in the face of evidence pointing out the inconsistency. But that does not commit us to calling her unhealthy *because she is unable to do the impossible.* Rather, we would just have to say that she is not well because she has inconsistent goals. The degree of ill health would depend on how serious the contradiction is and how dearly she holds onto it.

This is intimately connected with the fact that it is part of how we ordinarily understand what it means to intend to do something, what it means to set something as a goal for ourselves, that intentions connect and interact with beliefs in a coherent way.[9] This is the basis of so-called folk or belief-desire psychology. When someone seems to hold firmly to goals that are obviously logically incompatible, it becomes difficult to say that he or she really holds these goals at all. Instead, it seems that the individual suffers from a cognitive disorder. Such might be the case for a man who fully intends both to eat the piece of cake in front of him and to have that piece of cake remain intact on the plate for him to admire. Inconsistencies, even logical ones, need not be obvious, however. Where they are hidden, an individual might fail to see them without thereby being irrational or exhibiting a disorder.

A life plan might be inconsistent without being logically contradictory. Some goals are incompatible not logically but only due to contingent facts about how the world works. For instance, a voter in the United States might want to register as a Democrat in the state of Pennsylvania and vote in the Republican primary in New Jersey. Another person might have the goals of living without pain and of avoiding all visits to the dentist. These goals are not logically inconsistent, but they are generally incompatible in practice. Again, if a woman seems to understand the incompatibility of her goals and yet holds onto them quite strongly, without ranking them by priority or putting one aside, she will be unhealthy and may be diagnosed with a disorder.

It is to be expected, however, that many of us have goals that are in fact incompatible although we do not fully believe them to be so. The question remains as to which goals are the ones that count when assessing the health of such individuals. To address this question, I turn to the notion of an ideal observer. The relevant ideal observer would be a theoretical, rational version of the person who is able to sort through inconsistencies while maintaining the individual's core wants and values. I have in mind the ideal observer theory of ethics offered by Peter Railton.

Railton suggested the notion of an *objectified subjective interest* for an individual. These interests are determined by the facts about each person as suggested by the following thought experiment:

Give to an actual individual A unqualified cognitive and imaginative powers, and full factual and nomological information about his physical and psychological constitution, capacities, circumstances, history, and so on. A will have become A+, who has complete and vivid knowledge of himself and his environment, and whose instrumental rationality is in no way defective. We now ask A+ to tell us not what *he* currently wants, but what he would want his non-idealized self A to want—or, more generally, to seek—were he to find himself in the actual condition and circumstances of A. (Railton 1986, 173–74)

We might use this notion by saying that the goals we must consider when determining what constitutes health for an individual A are those that the corresponding idealized version of A, A+, would choose for A—A's objectified subjective interest. Idealizations are not what we are after in practical settings; however, in problematic cases we can use an idealized version of the individual in one of two ways. We can use it as a guide in making decisions on the patient's behalf; we can also set as a goal for education to bring each patient A closer to being an A+ so that she herself can revise her goals into a coherent and reasonable life plan.

(d) The final item on Nordenfelt's list of troubles for SG theories is the restricted applicability of the theory. He saw this as applying only to adult humans. The SG theory seems to have nothing to say about those too young to have their own goals for their lives, yet surely there is something to say about whether a given infant is healthy. Obviously, the Richman–Budson theory does not have this problem. There will always be an answer as to whether an infant is healthy qua organism. Furthermore, I do not think that judging the health of an infant qua person is as problematic as Nordenfelt suggested. Just as the very young depend on others to act on their behalf, so they must depend on others to set goals for them. The issue, although complicated, is no more complicated in the one case than in the other. Parental goals can serve as proxy for personal goals just as parental actions serve as proxy for personal actions of those too young to set goals and act for themselves. These proxy goals can thus be used to assess health of a child as a person until the time that he is able to form goals of his own.[10]

Problems with Goals: More Problems

With the addition of the strategy of conceiving an idealized version of the self (or patient) to be applied as outlined above, the Richman–Budson theory is able to address the problem cases raised by Nordenfelt quite adequately. Unfortunately, Nordenfelt's worries do not exhaust the dimensions on which the Richman–Budson theory needs clarification. Other issues are that some of our goals seem simply unrelated to health; that sometimes appropriate therapy involves revising goals themselves rather than adjusting a patient's abilities, and our theory does not at present seem to enable us to tell these cases from others; and that patients may have different personal goals during treatment and when not treated (cf. Nordenfelt 1994a, 182–83). I will address each of these in turn; treatment of each is developed further as the discussion unfolds in coming chapters. When we address the practical issues of deciding on recommendations for treatment we will consider the additional issue of the possible incommensurability of the goals of the individual qua person and the goals of the individual qua organism.

When we consider the health of individuals qua persons, we are faced with the fact that people have all sorts of goals that seem to have nothing to do with health. We have intuitions about what constitutes relevant goals—walking up stairs without pain, reproducing, and sleeping restfully are clearly related to health. They seem like relevant things to discuss with one's physician. But what about the goal of finding a four-leaf clover in my backyard? This might be indicative of ill health were it held firmly to the point of obsession or if my backyard were a concrete parking lot, but held moderately it seems to be neither here nor there with respect to the health of the individual who holds it.

Let us begin by thinking about goals that we understand to be problematic due to ethical rather than health concerns. We do not feel comfortable saying that the health care professional's (HCP's) role includes helping unethical people do morally reprehensible things, although it is clear that some persons have such actions among their goals. Morally reprehensible goals would include ridding the neighborhood of some ethnic group and causing pain to small children.[11]

One approach is to help the person *reinterpret* a problematic goal. For instance, a man may come to a clinic reporting that he wants to kill himself or someone else. After conversation, he may agree to a reinterpretation; his goal is acceptably restated as to stop the pain, or not to feel afraid or alone any more. Such reinterpretations bring the goal away from what is ethically problematic. Where no such reinterpretation is available or acceptable to the person, we may simply have an immoral patient. In these cases it will be clear what constitutes health of the individual; the question then becomes whether it is morally permissible to make such a man healthy. The moral status of a person's goals is not relevant to health as such.

An important issue remains, however; that is, when to initiate a strategy of reinterpretation. Surely professionals will be more likely to do that for goals of which they disapprove.[12] The problem of goal clarification will continue to engage our attention as this book progresses.

Body dysmorphic disorder (BDD) may be another condition in which reinterpretation of goals, perhaps through cognitive therapy, is the most appropriate way to restore health. A patient suffering from BDD believes that his or her body, which in fact falls under parameters usually considered normal and acceptable, is misshapen. Such individuals have the goal of changing the shape of their bodies. When surgery is denied or seems unavailable, it is not uncommon for them to resort to self-mutilation either in an attempt to perform the surgery themselves or to ensure that surgery becomes acceptable to their physicians (Highfield 2000).[13]

In early 2000 BDD came to the attention of the public in Britain after reports such as this one:

A Scottish hospital came under fire last week after it was revealed that one of its surgeons, Robert Smith, had done single-leg amputations on two physically healthy individuals with psychiatric disorders. "I have no doubt that what I was doing was the correct thing for those patients," Smith said. (Ramsay 2000)

On January 31, 2000, Dr. Smith, who is on staff at Falkirk & District Royal Infirmary, released a statement explaining that the patients suffered from apotemnophilia, which is a form of body dysmorphic disorder causing a desire to be an amputee. Smith explained that the patients had been given psychiatric and psychological assessments and, "Following amputation, they both made a rapid and satisfactory recovery without complications. At follow-up both patients remain delighted with their new state" (Ramsay 2000).

Smith's statement that the patients were "delighted with their new state" is especially challenging. Most of us, even those not particularly committed to the natural law approach to medical ethics and its associated principle of totality,[14] are at least a bit uncomfortable with the claim that the amputations were appropriate for these patients. Few will begrudge these people their delight, yet our discomfort with their decision seems more than just aesthetic. The Richman–Budson theory allows us to articulate the difficulty: we are made uncomfortable by these cases precisely because they highlight an apparent conflict between the health of the patients as persons and the health of the patients as organisms.[15]

However, studies have shown that surgery to make a BDD patient's body conform to a desired shape is in fact not reliably effective in helping the patient become satisfied. Quoting from a study by British psychiatrist David Veale, Ashraf (2000) wrote:

"Most patients . . . had multiple concerns about their appearance and reported that after 50% of the procedures the preoccupation transferred to another part of the body" . . . Even if surgery resolved a BDD problem, patients were still "significantly handicapped" by newfound complaints. (2055)

Although it seems to be typical of the human experience to be somewhat disappointed when we get things we have long wanted, the shifting preoccupation of BDD sufferers suggests that changing their bodies is not what these people really want. Indeed, more success has been seen with cognitive therapy to alleviate the preoccupation and thus remove the desire to change the body than has been seen with surgery (Geremia 1998). Cognitive therapy effects a change in the patients' desires by causing them to relinquish the judgment that their bodies are defective. (Note again the important interplay between beliefs and desires mentioned in our discussion of those with inconsistent goals.) Patients become less distressed, less depressed, and less anxious when they experience a reduction in the frequency and variety of these judgments. They are in effect accepting a reinterpretation of their original goal: they have accepted *being satisfied with their bodies* in place of *changing their bodies.*

This clarification of goals allows health care professionals (HCPs) to identify options available for bringing a patient closer to fulfilling these goals. In the case of BDD, cognitive therapy seems preferable to surgery not only because it is more reliably effective in reducing distress but also because as an attempt to improve the health of the individual qua person it is more consistent than surgery with the health of the individual qua organism. For some physicians, BDD sufferers whose goal of changing their bodies is intransigent are considered to pose an ethical dilemma. This may be especially true for physicians committed to the Catholic tradition of natural law ethics. For other physicians, such patients can be seen to generate a conflict between the health of the person qua organism and qua person. We will discuss how HCPs might deal with this conflict in parts II and III of this book.[16]

So far we have considered the effect of adjusting patient goals; however, as we have seen, changing a patient's beliefs can be just as important. We can understand the change effected in patients with BDD by cognitive therapy as primarily a change in belief rather than an affective change concerning which goals the patients desire to fulfill. These persons are described as having false beliefs. Diagnostic criteria for BDD begin with "A preoccupation with an imagined [*sic*] defect in appearance" (*DSM IV–TR* 2000, 510). Notably, the *DSM IV–TR* distinguishes between BDD and avoidant personality disorder/social phobia, the latter occurring in the presence of *actual* defects in appearance. Difficulties assessing personal appearance are legion. However, the *DSM IV–TR* confirms the suggestion that addressing treatment to a patient's beliefs can be as effective as addressing the patient's goals in creating an appropriate relationship between the two. Indeed, when people with BDD are unable to relinquish belief in the imagined defect even when faced with substantial evidence to the contrary, they may be given the additional diagnosis of "delusional disorder—somatic type" (*DSM IV–TR* 2000, 510).

Let us return to goals. The goal-reinterpretation approach is promising, as it involves pursuit of the real goals that may motivate the way a patient describes himself or herself to the HCP. We do not want to decide whether or how to treat an individual based on a too-quick assessment. However, implementing this approach requires that HCPs decide which reported goals should be reinterpreted. Moreover, highlighting the fact that patients can lack insight into their goals has dangers, not least that it could give professionals inappropriate confidence in reinterpreting those goals without appropriate dialogue. Consider also that an individual might simply want to kill or perform some other act that we may want to prevent. In this case it would be incorrect, even dangerous, to encourage the individual to assent to a reinterpretation of this goal. It is clear, however, that some otherwise unaccountable, unacceptable, or seemingly irrelevant goals can be removed from the picture by minimizing false beliefs.

Consider again the goal of finding a four-leaf clover. Suppose that I hold this goal. I do not spend my days examining lawns everywhere I go, but should I find myself among the right sort of vegetation I might spend a few moments looking, and in quieter times—perhaps while on vacation with my wife—I might say something such as, "Honey, don't you think it would be great to find a four-leaf clover? I've always wanted to do that." To reinterpret this goal, even to pay it much mind at all, would be to take it too seriously. I certainly see no need to discuss it with my HCPs. So what role does this goal play in determining my health? What are we to do with it? Where does it fit into the Richman–Budson theory? Our intuitions tell us that the fact that this goal is not a central part of my life plan is part of why I should not be considered unhealthy due to my (hitherto) inability to satisfy this goal. Another part of why failure to satisfy this goal does not make me unhealthy is the fact that I *could strive for* this goal should I decide to do so—I have the ability to find clover and to count the leaves on clover I see. Our sense of which goals deserve attention from HCPs will develop as the discussion continues.

Embedded instrumentalist accounts emphasize equilibrium, or match, between goals and abilities. We have articulated this as reach or strive for. In some cases health may be improved either by adjusting the goals or by adjusting the individual's abilities. I have mentioned cases in which the answer is clear as to which side of the equation it is appropriate to adjust. For someone whose goals include unaided flight, it is clear that the adjustment ought to be in the goals; for a person who is unable to breathe without pain, the adjustment ought generally to be in the abilities. In many cases, however, it is not immediately clear which side to adjust. Some of these cases arise in the context of rehabilitation medicine and disability, so I will discuss these briefly before begging the reader to accept yet another promise that the issues will seem less problematic as the discussion develops.

Rehabilitation is sometimes understood as the process of restoring an individual's abilities to normal, or to a level at which the person can return to work or live independently. This way of understanding rehabilitation may not be adequate for all patients, however:

> . . . using the word 'restoring', assumes that at some time in his life the patient has lived and worked 'normally' . . . But rehabilitation is concerned with many people who would not fall within the definition. (Stewart 1985, 1)

Stewart identified people who have been disabled from birth and the mentally handicapped as among those falling outside the definition. In addition, individuals may become permanently disabled. A professional basketball player who suffers a knee injury may have to be rehabilitated in order to learn to use the knee again and return to the game safely. If lucky, she may become healthy and achieve physical and vocational rehabilitation by improving her abilities. Should a professional basketball player become blind, however, she cannot return to her career. If she is lucky, she will find a way to adjust her goals in ways that are fulfilling and fulfillable.

In short, sometimes it is appropriate for goals to change. They may be adjusted downward, as athletic goals with age or after an injury. This allows us to say things such as, "Sam is mentally retarded and perfectly healthy," and "Maria is a healthy amputee." Given the separation of health and ethics, in a great many cases either adjusting goals or adjusting abilities will be equally effective at improving health of the patient qua person. The distinction between health and quality of life then takes on the job of accounting for why one move seems more desirable than the other. This distinction is addressed in chapter 3.

The last problem with goals that I will discuss here arises when an individual seems to have two sets of personal goals. Consider, for instance, a man who is in immediate need of dental care for which adequate anesthesia is unavailable. Before the pain begins, he may earnestly consent to the treatment. Once the pain becomes intense, he may begin to hold dearly to the goal of having the pain (and hence the treatment) stop immediately. Or consider the depressed patient who wants to die when not medicated and wants to live when medicated.[17] This phenomenon may be expected often with patients suffering from mood disorders or conditions for which treatment or lack of treatment causes intense discomfort. The question is whether preference ought to be given to one set of personal goals over another in such situations.

We can think about such cases by treating them as special instances of applying advance directives. Consider the last will and testament, generally a sort of financial advance directive. It has been traditional to begin a last will and testament with the words "I, [insert name], being of sound mind. . . ." This phrase is intended to differentiate between the goals made by the individual while sound of mind and those made by the same individual when impaired. However, this is not so easily accomplished without understanding what it means to be impaired. And it will seem well nigh impossible to assess whether an individual's stated intentions emerge from a state of health when we conceive of the intentions (goals) as *determining* what counts as health for that individual. As we have seen, it would be too easy to assume that an individual is of sound mind whenever her personal goals cohere with her goals as an organism. People can be of sound mind and decide to donate a kidney or use birth control. Individuals of sound mind might even choose to die in certain situations, for political or religious reasons, or to save someone else. So what are we to do? How can we determine which goals, intentions, or plans to honor when an individual articulates desires that, although not themselves inconsistent, are different from those articulated by the same individual in other circumstances? The answer lies, I believe, at the very core of the concept of autonomy as it has been developed in philosophical ethics. The issue of autonomy will occupy us quite a bit in the chapters to follow, so here I want only to offer a prolegomenon, as it were, to our future discussions.

Our everyday notion of autonomy involves self-determination, the ability to make choices for oneself. The philosophical understanding of autonomy is both more specific and more literal. It has its *locus classicus* in Kant's *Foundations of the Metaphysics of Morals*:

There is . . . only one categorical imperative. It is: Act only according to that maxim by which you can at the same time will that it should become a universal law. (Kant 1959, 39)

This first formulation of the categorical imperative offers a literal understanding of what it is to be auto-nomous–it is to give oneself laws, to be *sui juris*. Note that in this picture autonomy involves not just random independent actions, but *laws*. Laws are universal and hence issue in consistent patterns of behavior. No one who exhibits unconnected, irregular behavior is truly exercising autonomy in this literal, theoretical sense.

This understanding of autonomy underlies the widely accepted tenet according to which consent (to treatment, to participate in a research study, etc.) is accepted as informed and autonomous when it is consistent with other decisions the individual has made. This is precisely how the concept of autonomy can help us to think about our current issue. When an individual has expressed two different sets of goals or values, we can determine which to honor by looking for patterns in the person's past decisions. Should no such patterns be evident, it may be that the individual is not properly called autonomous. As Kant intended, this notion of autonomy coheres with a particular notion of rationality. When a patient is not autonomous, paternalism is called for. But more on autonomy and paternalism later.

Striving for Goals

Earlier I remarked that Whitbeck's theory shares an important element with the Richman–Budson theory that is missing from some other embedded instrumentalist theories: both allow that an individual may be healthy without being able to reach all of his or her goals. This allows for a life in which people are challenged to engage and hope for improvement. The Richman–Budson requirement of being able to strive toward satisfying goals is intended to be stronger than Whitbeck's requirement that the individual be able to respond in a way that is "supportive of" goals. Nordenfelt (1995) noted that an individual in poor health could make movements appropriate to and supportive of a goal and still be very far from reaching that goal. "Striving" is meant to capture something more than mere support. Showing up for the race is supportive of winning; to strive one must be *in* the race.

Note that someone could *be able to* reach or strive for a goal without ever actually reaching or striving for it. My goals include jitterbugging when the appropriate music is playing in the presence of an appropriate partner, and walking away when I am confronted by a barking dog. I may have the abilities appropriate for these goals even if I never again find myself in the relevant situations.

The specification that health is the ability to reach or strive for one's goals could be misleading. No one will be healthy who is able only to strive for goals without reaching any. However, our goals tend to be related to one another such that there are some that we would not be able to strive for unless we were able to reach others. One could hardly strive to run a marathon without being able to run a mile. We could not run a mile were we not able to walk, breathe, and satisfy all sorts of other goals. Similarly, one could not be a successful opera singer without being able to hear one's own voice. So it seems that a reasonable set of compatible goals tends to be such that if we are to *be able to reach or strive for* each goal, it must be the case that we are *able to reach* many of them. It does not seem analytic or otherwise necessary that our goals be related in these ways, but it does seem usual and likely that at least most are.[18]

Environmental Factors

The final issue that we will explore in this chapter is the role played by the individual's environment. Both in its social and physical aspects the environment can affect a person's ability to succeed in reaching his or her goals.

Nordenfelt (1995) described ability as a three-place relation among "the agent involved," "the goal of this agent," and "the circumstances in which the agent acts" (206). With this in mind, he observed that ability can change in response to changes in any of the three terms:

One way [that change in ability and hence health may come about] is a change in the biology or psychology of the person—for instance, the person may contract a disease which makes him or her unable to do what he or she was previously able to do. Another way is a change in the goals of the person: the person may develop new goals which are not realizable given the prevailing conditions. A third way is that the circumstances may change—for instance may become much harsher so that the agent is no longer able to realize all his or her goals. (207)

This all seems right. However, I suggest that the agent's environment need not be considered a separate issue when considering health of the agent qua person. Instead, we can consider the environment in which a goal is to be sought as part of the goal itself.

When I give my students a surprise quiz, it is generally understood that I intend them to complete it in the classroom in relative silence, and that each student should do his or her own work. The environment is not so much a separate factor but part of the assignment. Occasionally students have special needs, and for them the environment in which the quiz is to be taken is specified more explicitly. However, even then the conditions under which the task is to be completed need not be specified in their entirety. Environmental factors are implied by the goal itself and do not require specification. Bob wants to be able to walk to the store without an oxygen tank. We do not need to say that he wants to be able to do this on Earth rather than on the moon.

An individual may adopt the goal of living under the sea in an octopus's garden in the shade. If this is incompatible with other goals or with facts about what is possible in this world, the problem is not one of environment, but of the goals chosen or of the individual's beliefs. According to Nordenfelt, when we judge someone to be disabled, we usually do not need to specify an environment because the judgment comes in the context of background beliefs about what constitutes the relevant environment.[19] These background beliefs imply normative limitations, said Nordenfelt, and are often generated by societal standards. It seems to me that treating environmental limitations as a separate term only makes for a more complicated theory. Obviously, there is room for disagreement as to whether this complication is worth the cost.

What of the environment and health of the individual qua organism? Our bodies have developed for survival within certain parameters, including the composition of gases around us, the strength of gravitational forces to which we are subject, and so on. As we saw in our discussion of mild ADHD, individuals may be more or less well suited to particular variations within these parameters.[20] Some environments are clearly outside the range for which our bodies have developed. For instance, our bodies cannot be said to have the goal of breathing under water or in space, and we would not be called unhealthy for our inability to do these things. Conversely, our bodies can be said to have the goal of surviving in an environment in which we occasionally encounter pathogens that cause the common cold, and those who cannot survive exposure to such pathogens are unhealthy. But do the environments we are intended to survive in include those in which HIV is present? Our theory does not help us answer questions about marginal environments. There may be situations in which we are unable to determine whether we are, qua organisms, unhealthy or merely unlucky.[21]

It bears mentioning that the environment that serves as, in Nordenfelt's words, "a platform for action" (1994b, 36) includes not only the climate and available material resources, but also the interpersonal environment. Relationships, family support, social services, etc. all affect how individuals can implement their abilities.

Conclusion

Our discussion has developed a theory that ties the health status of individuals to the goals of those individuals. Individuals do not exist in a vacuum but in groups, and groups may themselves have goals. Such goals might be understood to ground a notion of social or public health. In addition, health care activities often occur in the contexts of a health care system and the medical profession. Both system and profession may also have goals. No doubt these goals also have to be recognized and dealt with, perhaps changed, to implement our theory. Although these broader issues must be acknowledged, we have quite enough to keep us busy as we grapple with our theory of health of individuals.

Our theory can be summarized as follows. An individual A is in a state of health when A is able to reach or strive for a consistent set of goals actually aimed at by A. Where A's goals are inconsistent in ways inaccessible to A, the relevant set of goals is that determined by the (idealized) objectified subjective interest of *A*. *A* will be unhealthy when false beliefs are central to *A*'s most firmly held goals. When we examine *A* as a biological organism, we find goals that may be incompatible with those *A* adopts as a conscious agent with plans for his or her life. Rather than try to adjudicate between these sets of goals, we embrace the conclusion that there may be two answers as to whether a given state is healthy for *A*. That is, we allow the possibility of conflict between the health of *A* qua organism and the health of *A* qua person.

This theory entails that there is a fact of the matter about what counts as healthy for people with clear goals predicated on primarily true beliefs, and acknowledges that these facts are often difficult to determine. If healthy states can vary as widely as individual goals, HCPs are obligated to discuss goals with each patient. And surely this sounds right—a fashion model and a professional athlete would rightly make different choices when deciding between a strength-restoring surgery to fix an injured knee and another procedure that would leave smaller scars, and we would not say that one choice led to a state that was intrinsically less healthy than the other. Our embedded instrumentalist theory can explain how the model's choice and the athlete's choice can both be healthy. It has the added virtue of helping us to explain how the healthy choice for a person can change from one stage of life to another (as in the case of a woman whose goals change to include pregnancy), or even from day to day (as in the case of Witty Ticcy Ray).

The most important conclusion to be drawn is that talking to patients about their goals is an absolutely central part of responsible health care. Medical science and biology may discover the means to reach our personal goals, but they tell us little about what those goals are or should be. For this reason, physicians and other HCPs cannot know what will improve the health of any individual considered as a person without substantial information about that individual's goals. This is worth emphasizing—the most competent HCP *cannot know what would count as healthy* for the patient qua person before gathering a great deal of information about the patient's individual concerns. This is not due to ethical worries about patient autonomy, but to metaphysical issues surrounding what it means to be healthy.[22]

Whereas the present work develops a justification and theoretical underpinning for this conclusion, it should be recognized that many physicians are already extremely sensitive to the significance of patient goals, especially in the context of end of life issues. For instance,

...as a matter of routine, physicians should become acquainted with their patients' personal values and wishes and should document them just as they document information about medical history, family history, and sociocultural background. Such discussions and the resultant documentation should be considered a part of the minimal standard of acceptable care. The physician should take the initiative in obtaining the documentation and should enter it in the medical record. (Wanzer et al. 1989, 845)

Pediatric orthopedic surgeons at Brigham and Women's Hospital in Boston also made explicit the importance of paying attention to patient goals. For example, when a patient has a tumor for which surgery is almost certainly appropriate, some physicians prescribe two or three months of chemotherapy. The express purpose is to get to know the patient and family so that the most appropriate solution can be found (Innovative Therapies . . . 2000, A4). The present discussion helps to justify precisely this "getting to know you" approach. Learning the patient's goals is an integral pair of determining what is healthy for the patient.

Another important conclusion is that cognitive therapy should be considered for individuals with apparently unrealistic, self-defeating, or inappropriate goals. Cognitive therapy addresses itself directly to beliefs rather than feelings in order to help people experiencing various kinds of distress:

Current cognitive therapies . . . hold in common these fundamental assumptions: that behavior and affect are mediated by cognitive processes; and that the task of the therapist is to identify these cognitions and to provide learning experiences which will modify them. Proponents of the cognitive therapies contend that correction of maladaptive cognitions will lead to improvement in psychiatric disorders. (Beck and Greenberg 1996, 230)

Our discussions of unrealistically high, inappropriately low, and incompatible goals suggested that these may in part be the result of "maladaptive cognitions" in the form of false beliefs. Beck, in particular, developed cognitive therapy techniques to help patients suffering from depression, panic disorder, and other problems identify false beliefs that keep them from setting and reaching reasonable goals.

These conclusions indicate how the theoretical theses developed here connect to ethical theory and clinical practice. The connections are developed in the chapters that follow. In part II we will see how our theory brings the goal of improving the health of patients qua persons into convergence with requirements for respecting patient autonomy.

II
Health and Ethics

3

Beneficence and Recommendations for Treatment

In this chapter I explore the status of the Richman–Budson theory as a theory of health. When I say that it is a theory of health, I mean that it allows us to sort individuals as they are at a given time into those who are healthy and those who are unhealthy. It also allows us to rank states of individuals as more or less healthy than other possible states of the same individuals. This theory tells us that health is indexed to goals, goals of organisms on the one hand for determining the health status of individuals qua organisms, and goals of moral agents on the other for determining the health status of individuals qua persons. The status of our theory as a theory of health is significant and subtle. It is one thing to honor an individual's goals out of simple respect for his or her autonomy, and another thing to recognize that examining these goals is necessary in order to establish whether the individual is healthy to begin with.

This distinction is worth drawing out. One reason to honor the wishes of individuals is that we believe that they have the right, ceteris paribus and within limits, to self-determination. Each person should be allowed to decide how his or her life goes. This is an ethical matter that affects the delivery of health care. In most theories of health, conscious decisions, the intentions or life plans of patients, are valued primarily for ethical reasons that are separated from specifically medical ones.

In the Richman–Budson theory, things are quite different. The theory states that facts about patient goals directly affect the health care professional's (HCP's) duty to benefit the patient. This duty falls under the principle of beneficence, which states that HCPs have an obligation to do good, to benefit their patients. This obligation is specifically directed at health-related goods. Thus if goals determine what will make individuals healthy, HCPs who are not thoughtful about these goals are in danger not just of failing to respect patient autonomy, but of failing in their duty of beneficence.[1] I do not want to suggest that most physicians make treatment decisions and suggestions without considering patients' goals and values. I maintain only that currently accepted theory and guidelines in medical ethics do not require that physicians consider these goals and values to the appropriate extent or for all of the right reasons.

This chapter addresses the issue of beneficence and treatment recommendations in the context of the Richman–Budson theory of health. For now, we consider only cases in which the goals of the individual are relatively clear and not counterproductive.

The Aims of Medicine

Ultimately, the import of our projects in this chapter concerns how to sort health care encounters into successful and unsuccessful ones, and to assess outcomes and processes by degrees of success in improving or sustaining the health of individuals. We want to be able to say something about the relative merits of past and completed health care encounters and of encounters currently competing for consideration. I have not said much directly on this topic so far. However, in the background of our discussions has been the reasonable (but perhaps naïve and insufficiently well-formed) idea that the success of an encounter is to be assessed according to whether the patient is closer to perfect health for having been involved than he or she would otherwise have been.

In my account, an encounter can be successful with respect to both the individual qua organism and the individual qua person, with respect to only one of these, or with respect to neither. Comparison of alternative treatments falls out along the same lines: treatment A would be more successful than treatment B if the patient would be more healthy for having pursued treatment A than she would have been for having pursued treatment B. As with the assessment of interventions considered singly, comparative assessments may diverge along the organism-person fault line, so that A may be better than B for the health of the patient qua organism but worse than B with respect to the health of the patient qua person. I do not claim that we will always be able to determine that a given option is better, worse, or equivalent to a certain other option, but without some sense of how we might compare options, a theory of health would be empty.

This picture of the goals of health care is open to criticism along several lines. One might object that improving health is not the only goal, that health care encounters of an individual should not be assessed one at a time, or that they should not be assessed by considering only one individual at a time. One might also protest the narrow focus on outcomes rather than processes, or the way the given account isolates the patient from the HCP rather than recognizing the importance of the professional-patient relationship.

Whereas these are all reasonable objections, I plead immunity to them in this chapter. It seems correct to claim that improving health of individuals is not the only goal of health care encounters; HCPs face moral and social issues that obligate them, and economic goals may also rightly play a role. Issues of the relationship between patient and HCP are included in these sorts of obligations. We addressed some general issues concerning the relationship between health and ethics in chapter 2. In a broader picture, it may turn out that improving the health of one individual would be a bad thing, or worse than an alternative course of action. However, for now we consider only the good that we might do for individuals considered by themselves and on their own terms, and primarily as regards their health.

We are fortunate to live in a world in which the goals of individual persons often encompass the interests of others. For many people, their goals specify how they want to help others, so that consideration of the health of an individual will not be quite as individualistic as may seem. Of course, we have no guarantee that this will be the case. We may find ourselves facing a situation in which improving the health of one individual will contribute to injustice or be immoral for other reasons. That this will not change the medical character of the situation does not mean that medicine is beyond the scope of morals.

Because our theory of health is concerned with the goals of individuals, it is forward-looking and takes into account the future states of the individual. Thus, my formulation of how we might assess health care encounters builds in concern for the relationship between one encounter and those to come. This feature avoids an undue focus on outcomes in terms of the resultant state of the individual rather than the process of providing health care—a single encounter will increase the health of a patient only if it contributes to a (relatively) long-term plan. Other issues regarding process, such as those related to informed consent, are ethical concerns that, although critical to health care in general, are peripheral to our immediate project.

We still have to take a quick peek at some other ways of specifying the goals of medical encounters to be sure that we do not miss anything. The following characterization of the goals of medicine coheres well with mine: "... the function of medicine is to preserve autonomy," and "preservation of life is subservient to the primary goal" (Cassell 1977, 18). Borrowing from Gerald Dworkin, Cassell explained that autonomy requires independence and authenticity of self. Illness reduces both of these. Reduced independence means reduced freedom to act on one's choices; reduced authenticity, a state in which the patient is not her "true" self, reduces the likelihood that her stated preferences cohere with her more considered, underlying goals and values. This emphasis on goals and abilities makes Cassell's account consistent with, even akin to, my account of the goals of medical care.

In 1993, the Hastings Center began a research project entitled the Goals of Medicine. The consensus document resulting from this project identified four goals:

(1) the prevention of disease and injury and the promotion and maintenance of health; (2) the relief of pain and suffering caused by maladies; (3) the care and cure of those with a malady, and the care of those who cannot be cured; and (4) the avoidance of premature death and the pursuit of a peaceful death. (Hanson and Callahan 1999, xi)

The definition of health they offer in conjunction with these goals of medicine is a catch-all that raises rather than answers many of the questions we explored in part I.[2] In addition, the goals are specified in terms more global than those concerning individual encounters or even individual patients. Even so, they accord roughly with the gist of my commonsense understanding: medicine should aim to provide more of the health-related good stuff and help people avoid health-related bad stuff, essentially to increase health and decrease disease. We have seen that there are many ways of specifying what counts as health and as health related. Chapter 2 specified what I take to be the good and bad stuff that relate directly to health.

An important theme is the idea that "curing disease" is not an adequate specification of the goals of medical care. The Hastings Center report called for "Balancing the Curative Bias"[3] (Hastings Center 1999, 8). Pellegrino and Thomasma also rejected the idea that curing disease is the true goal of medical care, instead articulating it in terms of "healing." They defined the goal of medicine as "a right and good healing action for a particular patient" (Pellegrino and Thomasma 1988, 10). This action should address body-related aspects of disease and illness, as well as psychosocial aspects, and, as they put it, "spiritual dimensions" of the individual's condition:

To heal is to make whole or sound, to help a person reconvene the powers of the self and return, as far as possible, to his conception of a normal life. (Pellegrino and Thomasma 1988, 10)

Where Pellegrino and Thomasma wrote that "healing involves more than a cure," I have presented cases in which curing disease would worsen the patient's health qua person. Curing Witty Ticcy Ray's Tourette's syndrome, for instance, would keep him from reaching his musical goals. In the Richman–Budson theory, improvement of health becomes detached from curing diseases as traditionally understood.

Beneficence

Beneficence has not had much time in the spotlight of medical ethics. Bioethics has been rightly concerned with protecting patient autonomy, access to care, whether it is permissible to apply new genetic technologies, and other issues. Beneficence is also likely to be ignored as a principle guiding ethics because it may seem empty. It rings of a simplistic Bill and Ted approach to ethics: *be excellent to one another.* But there are important things to say about it.

William K. Frankena (1973) suggested that beneficence should be understood as central to our understanding of ethics in general. He proposed building our moral theory on two principles: beneficence and just distribution. According to Frankena, recognition that we have an obligation to do good combines with an understanding of how this good should be distributed to ground our moral judgments. Without an obligation to beneficence, no determination of what is good or right has a bearing on us.

Pellegrino and Thomasma emphasize that beneficence is important in addressing challenges left unanswered by conflicts between autonomy and paternalism:

Distinguished ethicists such as Childress recognize the . . . conflicts between autonomy and paternalism. They prefer to err, if they must, on the side of autonomy on what we consider erroneous metaethical grounds, namely that rights take precedence over goods. (Pellegrino and Thomasma 1988, 15)

Paying too much attention to the issue of who gets to decide (an issue of rights) can draw our attention away from what should be the central question of health care encounters: what will be best for the patient (an issue of goods)? This is especially clear in the light of Pellegrino and Thomasma's reminder that occasions on which important decisions are to be made are nearly always occasions when the patient's autonomy is impaired:

If we take the impact of illness and disease seriously, we must modify the autonomy model. That model has four features: self-direction, establishing a life plan, deliberating about applying a life plan (reasoning and information), and acting on the basis of such deliberations. (Pellegrino and Thomasma 1988, 17)

Poor health can affect all four of these features of autonomy. Beneficence then takes center stage over autonomy and paternalism as the guiding principle or value in the treatment of ill patients.[4]

The principle of beneficence is general and schematic, identifying no specific duty: it "is in general simply the principle of doing good" (Engelhardt 1996, 112). Engelhardt treated the community as the unit that determines what counts as beneficent. By "Expressing the principle of beneficence in the maxim 'Do to others their good' . . .", he meant their good in light of the view of the good life accepted by their community, not by the patient as an individual. The Richman–Budson theory of health makes it very clear that what constitutes medical benefit for each patient qua person will vary from person to person and not just community to community.

It is common in bioethics to distinguish between a principle of beneficence and a principle of nonmaleficence (often expressed in the famous dictum *primum non nocere*). Frankena treated them as one, and understood beneficence as follows:

What does the principle of beneficence say? Four things, I think:
1. One ought not to inflict evil or harm (what is bad).
2. One ought to prevent evil or harm.
3. One ought to remove evil.
4. One ought to do or promote good. (Frankena 1973, 47)

How is this to be applied in the context of medical care? Citing what he termed "*the samaritan principle*," Wulff (1995, 298) described ". . . a duty to help others in case of illness."[5] Speaking generally, this means that HCPs have a duty to be proactive; when opportunities arise to act in ways that will benefit a patient, an HCP has a prima facie duty to do so.[6] This duty will often be challenged by other prima facie duties involving just distribution of resources, as well as the prima facie duty to respect the patient's autonomy.

Physician Atul Gawande (1991) advocated beneficence ("kindness") over blind adherence to stated patient preferences. At times HCPs should be firm in leading a patient to make a medically appropriate decision, even when the patient, if left to his or her own judgment, would choose otherwise. Some see this attitude as impermissible because it is coercive and thus limits autonomy in favor of paternalism. Gawande, on the other hand, couched his point in beneficence talk: ". . . as the field grows ever more complex and technological, the real task isn't to banish paternalism; the real task is to preserve kindness." (91)

Like Pellegrino and Thomasma, Gawande recognized that patients, especially when ill, can fail to make decisions that are rational in the context of their own goals:

People are rightly suspicious of those claiming to know better than they do what's best for them. But a good physician cannot simply stand aside when patients make bad or self-defeating decisions—decisions that go against their deepest goals. (Gawande 1999, 88)

In this context, beneficence demands a weak form of paternalism; when the patient's perspective and abilities are compromised, the HCP must sometimes go against the patient's expressed preferences and act in ways that advance the patient's more settled goals.

My approach to ethics begins to emerge. This discussion shows my sympathy with moral principles such as beneficence and autonomy. These principles have their own theoretical and intuitive legitimacy, as well as serving to generalize and codify our assessments of what constitute appropriate actions in specific cases.[7] The concept of prima facie duty comes in because the duties entailed by principles in specific cases may conflict. Such conflicts do not show that the duties entailed are without force. These duties retain their force, but some are not acted on because they are trumped by others.

Beneficence and Quality of Life

Beneficence is especially important to discussions of quality of life. Quality of life has been used to assess the relative value of treating different conditions to determine the most effective distribution of health care, as a tool for clinicians facing difficult treatment decisions, and as a way of giving information to patients so that they can exercise autonomy (Häyry 1991, 97).

Facing difficult decisions concerning devastating diseases and debilitating treatments, clinicians and researchers often attempt to compare options in terms of quality (and length) of life the patient can expect on pursuing each option, sometimes specifying this in terms of expected *quality of life years* (QOLYs). The point of assessing treatments in terms of absolute and comparative expected quality of life is to make it more likely that the parties will choose a therapy that offers the greatest net benefit to the patient. Quality of life is not the same thing as health, but often depends on health at least in part. Before noting how the two differ, it will be useful to have an idea of what has been meant by quality of life.

In 1977, Anthony Shaw argued against the concept that quality of life is simply proportional to "quantifiable physical and mental characteristics." He constructed a formula to capture this conception of quality of life as follows:

$QL = NE$; *where* (QL) represents quality of life and (NE) represents the patient's natural endowment (physical and intellectual). (Shaw 1977, 11)

The formula suggests that, ceteris paribus, individuals who are stronger and/or smarter have a higher quality of life. This is simplistic, false, and vaguely offensive. It seems reasonable to claim that an individual with an IQ of 35 will have a lower quality of life than that same individual might have had with an IQ of 120.[8] However, it is not at all clear that that individual's life would continue to improve with each increase in mental capacity. There are decreasing marginal gains for intelligence, as exist for physical prowess, as well. Indeed, costs of being at the high end of any biostatistical measurement come with the fact that few others are similar. The lives of sideshow attractions such as the "strong man" or "human calculator" are not guaranteed to be more—or less—desirable than those of the average furniture mover or actuary.

It is interesting that Shaw's suggested revision of this conception does very little to remove what is distressing about it. He merely adds family and societal contributions, so that the revised formula reads:

$QL = NE \times (H + S)$ in which (H) represents the contributions made to that individual by his home and family and (S) represents the contributions made to that individual by society. (Shaw 1977, 11)

In this new formulation, it still comes out that, ceteris paribus, individuals who are stronger and/or smarter have a higher quality of life. He has only specified some of the *cetera* that can fail to be *paria*.

Philosophers define quality of life in three ways: first, *perfection*, that is, how well that person "realizes important human potentials"; second, "pleasure and absence of pain"; and third, "preference-satisfaction," or the degree to which "the person gets what he wants" (Sandøe 1999, 13). Each of these is a way of answering the question, "What makes a person's life go well?", and can serve as the basis for "three different views about the nature of the good life . . . *Perfectionism, Hedonism* and *the Preference Theory*." Sandøe notes that "In many real-life cases these views will deliver the same verdict about a person's quality of life" (Sandøe 1999, 13). Derek Parfit (1984) provided a similar taxonomy, distinguishing among "*Objective List Theories*," "*Hedonistic Theories*," and "*Desire-Fulfillment Theories*" of "what makes someone's life go best" (493).

Perfection is an Aristotelian view that relies on there being a fact about what comprise "important human potentials." This view shares some features with the Richman–Budson theory of health of individuals qua organisms.[9] Hedonism is akin to utilitarianism—troubling in its simplest form, but perhaps made more palatable by bells and whistles such as distinguishing, as did John Stuart Mill, between mere "swine" pleasures and the "higher" pleasures that make human lives most rich.

Preference-satisfaction views are more common in discussions of quality of life than in discussions of health as such. For instance,

A good quality of life can be said to be present when the hopes of an individual are matched and fulfilled by experience. The opposite is also true: a poor quality of life occurs when the hopes do not meet with the experience . . . (Calman 1984, 124–25)

This requires an individual's hopes to be realistic, and thus appropriate to his or her actual situation. Since each individual's situation changes through time, the person's hopes must also change. Obviously, the preference-satisfaction view shares much with the Richman–Budson theory of health of individuals qua persons. As with hedonism, difficulties that arise in the simple form of the preference-satisfaction view can be eschewed by making appropriately sophisticated clarifications, in this case, along the lines discussed in chapter 2.[10]

Häyry (1991) recognized definitions of quality of life based on needs and definitions based on wants. The needs view is driven by the desire for a scientific and objective standard, preferably involving observable and measurable data.[11] The wants view is what Sandøe called the preference-satisfaction view. As Häyry notes, the needs approach fails to incorporate "the subjective aspects of human life . . ."; on the other hand, the wants approach ". . . tends to ignore some of the objective realities of the human existence" (Häyry 1991, 97).

Häyry raised precisely the tension that led to our embracing both a theory of health of persons and a theory of health of organisms. Indeed, Häyry even addressed the issue of personal preferences and amputation, a topic that vexed us somewhat in chapter 2. Häyry (1991) separated the issue of quality of life from that of health:

. . . in quality-of-life assessments objective criteria such as state of health and observable behaviour must always, in the end, be submitted to the patient's own judgement. Amputation of a limb, for instance, obviously worsens someone's bodily condition, but the influence the operation has upon one's physical performance or enjoyment of life varies individually and over time. (105)

The idea seems to be that quality of life may be subjective and indexed to wants even if health turns out to be objective and more about needs. This notion of quality of life is much like the Richman–Budson notion of health of persons.

Instruments actually used to assess quality of life often include direct subjective questionnaires in which the patient is asked to rate quality of life on a numerical scale (1–10, e.g.) or indicate a level of agreement or disagreement with statements such as "my current quality of life is very high" using a Likert scale. A surrogate, such as a parent or caregiver, is surveyed for children and those incapable of producing appropriately considered answers themselves. Other instruments may be completed by an HCP on the basis of the patient's observable states or information collected for the patient's medical record.

Quality of life measurements were introduced in part to provide a subjective complement to measurements of health, which have been taken to be objective and value free. I contended that health has subjective components and that we do not and should not think of it as value free. In short, my way of understanding health is more like the usual ways of understanding quality of life than is, for example, Boorse's biostatistical theory of health. The Richman–Budson theory does not put quality of life out of business, however.

One way that health and quality of life can diverge is if an individual has abilities that cannot be exercised. A person could be endowed with abilities adequate for reaching or striving for reasonable, consistent, and even ethically permissible goals but be prevented from reaching many goals due to hostile environmental factors. Consider Joe and Jane. Joe is able to fulfill his goal of walking to the train station, but is kept from doing so by riot police suppressing revolutionaries on his block. Joe's wife, Jane, has all of the abilities required for achieving her goal of finishing a doctoral dissertation by December, but is unable to do so because, while returning from the library, she was arrested outside her apartment on suspicion of revolutionary activity. Given their goals, Joe and Jane have abilities that make them healthy, and yet have a poor quality of life because they are in an environment importantly different from the one implied by their goals. Quality of life is generally assessed with reference to goals of individuals qua persons, although it is often affected by reductions or improvements in ability to reach goals that we would intuitively attribute to the individual qua organism. A lower level of health, including a lower level of health of an individual qua person, in most cases results in a lower quality of life.

Richness

Preference-satisfaction views of quality of life are, of course, subject to the same objections as their parallel theories of health. In response to Calman's view, Häyry described a challenging case in which a physician is discussing alternative treatments with a patient. The physician recommends a radical and risky procedure and promises to restore quality of life afterward if adverse outcomes occur:

> In such a situation, the patient obviously has every right to assume that the physician refers to life-quality as the patient experiences it now, against the background of his present expectations and values. However, if one takes Calman's points seriously, all the doctor is saying is that *either* the patient's occurrent wishes can indeed be fulfilled even after the radical procedure, *or* they can be modified to match reality by persuasion and therapy. (Häyry 1991, 112)

The preference-satisfaction view suggests that if a treatment reduces a patient's abilities, the patient's quality of life can be restored equally fully by restoring his abilities *or* by lowering his goals to match his diminished abilities. This is clearly wrong. Something seems to be missing in naïve preference-satisfaction views.

In chapter 2 we paid special attention to Nordenfelt's embedded instrumentalist theory of health. Nordenfelt also endorsed a preference-satisfaction account of quality of life that is in accord with his theory of health, putting it in terms of "happiness with life"[12] (Nordenfelt 1994b, 38). He introduced a dimension of preference satisfaction that is absent from our discussion of health and that addresses the worry raised by Häyry. Nordenfelt called this dimension "richness." Enriching a person's set of goals is improving it in some sense, not just enlarging it. Take the example of P. As a young man, P starts out with expectations and goals:

[P] wishes to become a clerk in a bank like his father and starts working in the local branch of the national bank. His life fulfills all his modest expectations and ambitions. Thus P is completely happy in the equilibrium sense. Later, however, he is persuaded to set his goals higher. He starts an advanced course in banking and soon reaches a top position in his bank. As a result of this change he has become, as he also himself claims, much happier. Still, in the want-equilibrium sense, he was completely happy already from the beginning. (Nordenfelt 1994b, 53)

The claim here is that there are more and less rich sets of goals, and thus more and less rich ways of being happy. Having all of one's goals met is not always the best one can do.[13] It is clear that someone who is happy in a richer way has a higher quality of life.[14] The concept of richness captures the way in which the patient in Häyry's example might end up with a lower quality of life despite equilibrium between his goals and abilities.

The notion of richness also connects to the objection raised by Matthew Clayton, which we deferred dealing with in chapter 2. Clayton was concerned that Nordenfelt's embedded instrumentalist theory is prejudiced in favor of those with higher expectations (Clayton 1999, 63). If you and I have similar biological problems but I want more out of my life than you do, then, in my theory of health, it is likely that it will take more resources to make me healthy (qua person) than it will to make you healthy (qua person). When we see Clayton's objection in light of the fact that members of higher socioeconomic classes tend to have higher expectations for their lives (higher goals) than do members of less privileged groups, embedded instrumentalist theories may seem to excuse unfair distributions of health care.

I could respond by assimilating the issue into that of making sure that people are counseled to set appropriate and appropriately high goals. With this move I would deny that individuals with low goals are actually healthy, and group them with those who have inconsistent goals or goals based on false or unproductive beliefs.

I favor a second way of responding to Clayton's objection, in which we swallow the conclusion with respect to health and redescribe the issue in terms of quality of life. I allow that indeed it takes more resources to make a person with higher goals healthy than it does to make a person with lower goals healthy, but add the qualification that this is not the whole story. In their professional roles, HCPs have a prima facie duty to improve the health of their patients. However, in their role as fellow citizens, as human beings, and (perhaps) as educators, they may also have a duty to improve patients' quality of life. One way to perform this duty would be to help individuals adopt and realize richer sets of goals.

This second approach is consistent with the way I have been distinguishing between ethical issues and medical ones. Yes, it is morally repugnant that in our society those with socially inherited power and wealth are systematically trained to set higher goals in life. Yes, HCPs have as much obligation to do something about this as do others. But this obligation is not specifically health related or medical. Improving quality of life is as much the province of politicians, police officers, and teachers, to name a few, as of physicians and other HCPs.

That said, we are not always able to sort problems neatly into those of poor health and those of low quality of life, and for this reason it is impossible to say which we are aiming to improve in a given case. The question, "Am I encouraging higher goals in this individual to make her more healthy or to give her a richer quality of life?" need not be answerable in all cases. It is more important to improve the person's general situation than to determine whether one is acting on a specifically medical duty to improve health rather than the corollary duty to improve quality of life.

Even lumping together improvements in both quality of life and health, richness accounts such as Nordenfelt's can seem to give us the wrong answer in some cases. Derek Parfit suggested such a case in his discussion of "summative" preference-based theories. Summative theories rank states of individuals according to how many of a person's desires are fulfilled and how many are unfulfilled, weighting each desire according to the intensity with which it is held. Parfit asks us to consider a situation in which he causes an individual to become addicted to a drug, which he subsequently supplies in quantities sufficient to fulfill the strong and recurring desire. Summative theories must hold that Parfit has benefitted the person by increasing the number of desires being fulfilled and increasing the proportion of fulfilled versus unfulfilled desires. Of course, one desire, not to be a drug addict (or to be cured of the addiction), will not be fulfilled. But this desire would be well outweighed by "an indefinite series of extremely strong desires, one each morning," for the drug. And each of these desires will be satisfied because Parfit is supplying plenty of the addictive drug. "On the Summative Theories, by making you an addict, I will be benefiting you—making your life go better" (Parfit 1984, 497).

Parfit suggested that the summative theorist can avoid this implausible conclusion by appealing to our second-order desires through what he called global versions of the summative theories. Global theories consider the preferences we have for our lives considered holistically, including our preferences for what desires we might have. Considered this way, we can respond to the addiction example by noting that most people would prefer not to have the addict's desire, although they would prefer the desire to be satisfied should they have it.

But it is conceivable that someone *would* in fact prefer to have the addict's desire, especially if it is certain that it will be fulfilled. We respond that this kind of desire does not add richness to an individual's life even though certain other desires would. (Although Parfit rejected summative theories on different grounds, we can see that if certain values are enriching and others not, this gives us another reason to hold that naïve summative theories will not serve us well in quality of life assessments.)

Nordenfelt's story of the bank clerk suggests that richness really does make a difference in quality of life. But how might we sort desires into those that provide richness and those that do not? Is the lawyer's daily desire for an espresso machiatto enriching? The college student's weekly desire for beer and pizza? The connoisseur's desire for a good cigar? The Rastafarian's desire for ganja? The Elvis fan's desire to see the King in concert? Individuals with these desires will be poor judges of whether the desires enrich their lives so as to maximize their quality of life. Each desire can be strong and important in the lives of these individuals; but like Nordenfelt's young bank clerk, the individuals will not know what it is like to have different desires until they actually adopt them.

A difference does seem to exist between the child's desire for Hershey's Kisses and the adult's desire for fine Belgian chocolate that parallels the difference between the fraternity man's desire for beer and the connoisseur's desire for a good wine. We may want to explain our intuitions on this by noting the degree to which the intellect is engaged, or by distinguishing, with J. S. Mill, between higher pleasures and swine pleasures. Nordenfelt suggested a distinction between more and less "ambitious" goals. The difference may also be explained along the lines of Rawls's (1971) Aristotelian Principle by the way the connoisseur delights in improving his skill at discerning tastes and aromas. Also, some desires lead to behavior that is clearly unhealthy for individuals qua persons (e.g., a desire for violence) or qua organisms (e.g., a desire to smoke tobacco). However, neither of these seems a definitive tool for selecting enriching goals, and I see no reason to suggest that they would provide very similar assessments.

It looks as if our judgments concerning which desires are enriching and which not are determined largely by culture. This explains in part why it seems normal to say, "Sorry, I haven't had my morning coffee," but not, "Sorry, I haven't had my morning joint." It also explains certain aspects of American culture, such as outlawing marijuana while advertising whiskey on highway billboards. Of course, some cultural determinations are misled, as the American fascination with cigarettes turned out to be. If richness is a factor in quality of life (as it seems to be) and if it is determined in part by culture (as it seems to be), quality of life assessments must be made in the light of values concerning which desires are enriching, where these values may vary from community to community and in individual communities through time.

The role of culturally relative values in assessing quality of life is another way that health and quality of life diverge. Goals that are relevant to determinations of health are those of the individual alone; values that count in assessing richness in sets of goals for determining quality of life are those of a larger group.

Medicalizing Problems with Living and Distribution of Care

The Richman–Budson theory of health of individuals qua persons draws fire from those who distinguish between medical problems and other problems with living. In chapter 1 we saw that Thomas Szasz drew this distinction. From Szasz's perspective, our theory will seem to "medicalize" problems that are not truly medical. This can be used to set up objections such as Clayton's. Generally put, the objection is that pitching the medical tent to include every dissatisfaction with life is likely to direct resources to those with high ambitions, and that would be unjust because high ambitions often stem from general privilege to begin with.

Evaluating the health of individuals is skew to issues of justice. The medically best treatment for a patient can be outrageously costly, so that providing it is obviously out of the question for reasons of justice and resources. But that does not change what would be medically best for this individual if resources were not an issue. This would be true in nearly every theory of health of individuals.

To isolate the health of individuals is, of course, to abstract this issue from its conceptual and worldly context. Justice must play a part in how people are cared for in real-world situations. I have not promised a theory of just distribution of care, and do not plan to deliver one. However, I do want to suggest that it might be fruitful to consider issues of distributive justice with respect to health care in light of the preceding discussion of quality of life.

According to my exposition, health and quality of life are both matters of being able to reach or strive for goals. Quality of life is more affected by specific features of the environment that impede or enable exercise of an individual's abilities. In addition, it rises with richness of the goal set. Richness is assessed according to community standards, and sets containing few goals can be richer than those containing many goals. Justice is about distribution of goods among individuals, and health and quality of life are different but intertwined goods. Thus an approach to health care justice for a particular society might balance the two. For instance, a community might have enough resources to guarantee health care sufficient for a certain minimum quality of life (for all who are able to reach such a level). Probably this will leave many people unhealthy by virtue of wanting abilities the community cannot afford. But this would be a way to conceptualize a just distribution of health care.

Except when it involves goal enrichment, quality of life care generally improves the health of individuals qua persons. However, we will not find criteria for determining the just distribution of care within the concepts of health and quality of life themselves.

Deciding among Treatment Options

Patients and HCPs are often faced with situations in which any of several treatments or courses of action would be reasonable. Some of these situations involve economic choices. For example, one might consider whether it is worth paying more to have a plastic surgeon close a wound rather than a general surgeon in order to avoid a visible scar, or whether it is worth paying more for a prescription-strength drug when one could have partial relief from an over-the-counter product. These are cases of balancing the good of health against other goods. Such balancing is important and deserves attention, but is not part of our current project.

Here we have to consider two types of situations. In one type, a decision must be made among courses of action that would be equally healthy for the individual qua organism but in different ways, so that each could affect the health of the individual qua person differently. In the other case, a decision must be made, because what would improve the health of the individual qua person would diminish the health of the individual qua organism and vice versa.

In the first case, since the alternatives yield different levels of health qua person and the same level of health qua organism, the choice that best fulfills the duty of medical beneficence is the one that most improves the health of the individual qua person. This situation makes it perfectly clear how, in my theory of health, an HCP could be unable to determine how to act on a duty of beneficence in the fullest way due to lack of access to the patient's personal, individual goals.

When the HCP is able to work with the patient to set goals for care that match the patient's overall life goals, the decision can come into focus. Consider, for instance, a person with cancer for whom surgery and a combination of radiation and chemotherapy promise equal benefits and risks for health qua organism. If it is particularly important to this man to retain his hair, perhaps to enhance self-esteem or maintain social and business relationships, surgery might be healthier for that man qua person. If a woman has a particular fear of surgery, or holds to a religious prohibition against surgery or blood transfusions, nonsurgical treatment might be healthier. Physicians may be inclined to say of such situations that the choice is not a medical one at all, that it arises precisely because each option offers equal medical benefits. This is true when we consider only health of the patient qua organism. It is central to my position that such choices are not *just* a matter of personal preference, but that they make a real difference in the patients' health when we consider patients qua persons.

Some individuals with ADHD face a similar type of choice. Ritalin (methylphenidate) is commonly used to treat ADHD. It has few side effects, but some physicians worry that patients can develop tolerance to it and can become dependent on it.[15] To address the issue of dependence, access to Ritalin is controlled by requiring patients to obtain a new prescription each month. To address the issue of tolerance, patients can be advised to take the drug only five of every seven days. Given these restrictions, Ritalin will improve health of the patient qua organism a great deal, but can do the job only to a level approaching five-sevenths of what is required. Wellbutrin (bupropion) may also be used to treat ADHD. It does not carry a risk of tolerance or dependence and so may be taken seven days out of seven. However, it does increase risk of seizures. Thus, whereas Wellbutrin may address the poor function associated with ADHD more fully than restricted therapy with Ritalin, the accompanying risk makes it no more healthy for the patient qua organism. A choice between these options must be made on the basis of which will be better for the health of the patient qua person.

Other cases in this category involve clear trade-offs between or among goals. For instance, SSRIs (selective serotonin reuptake inhibitors), used to treat depression, can inhibit libido and sexual function. Both sexual function and serotonin levels (which regulate mood) are important to the health of human organisms, so that in many cases (although not all, e.g., not in the case of a suicidal depressed patient) improving one at the cost of the other may not make a difference in level of overall health qua organism. Here, too, the goals of the patient qua person should dictate the choice of treatment. Indeed, physicians sometimes recommend that patients lower the dosage of a given SSRI at times when sexual function is important. For instance, Professor East manages his depression with an SSRI. He lives quite far from his wife, Professor West, and they meet only when their institutions are both between terms. His sexual function is a much greater priority to him when they are together than when they are apart, and he may choose to adjust the balance between his mood and his sexual function accordingly.

Professor East's case may remind us of Witty Ticcy Ray, whom we discussed in chapter 2; however, the two are different in a very important way. For Ray, adjusting his medication made him less healthy qua organism. Professor East, on the other hand, chooses to balance mood and sexual function in a zero sum trade-off. Thus he chooses between states that are equally healthy for him qua organism to find the one that makes him most healthy qua person.

Another type of zero sum case comes about when a patient has limited resources and must choose how to allot them. A patient in need of extensive rehabilitation services, whose insurance and savings allow enough care to improve functioning in only a subset of related areas, may have to choose whether to work on cognitive skills, manual dexterity, or mobility. Here, too, several paths may be equally healthy for the patient qua organism, but will bring one level of goal satisfaction to a dance instructor and a different level to a mathematician. Indeed, studies show that real differences exist among patient groups (and between patient groups and professional groups) concerning which abilities are most valued (Stineman et al. 1998).

One cannot be blamed for failure to act on information that is unobtainable. For instance, in an emergency room when a patient arrives unconscious and unaccompanied, no information about the specific preferences of the patient qua person will be accessible. Decisions might be made in such situations that turn out not to have maximized the health of the individual qua person. However, in such situations, any choice that is good for the patient qua organism is permissible.

When the health of a patient qua person conflicts with the health of the patient qua organism, the choice of treatment can be much more unsettling for all involved. Many cases of apparent conflict will be resolvable along lines suggested in chapter 2. For instance, a woman suffering from anorexia may state that she wants to be thinner, but this desire may be relinquished through revision of a harmful false belief. Other cases will turn out to be about other kinds of choices. For instance, a mother with too little food for herself and her child may choose to postpone satisfying her own desire to eat so that her child can eat.

It can be difficult to separate personal goals from organism goals. Consider a decision that faced patients with torn anterior cruciate ligaments (ACLs) in their knees. Although new techniques have made the choice less stark, these patients at times were asked to choose between two surgical interventions. The first removes the torn ligament to avoid further damage to the knee. It causes minimal external scarring and leaves the knee at below normal strength and agility. The second surgical procedure reconstructs the ACL, leaving substantial external scarring and enabling recovery to near-normal function. (New surgical techniques allow ACL reconstruction with much smaller incisions and hence less scarring, but we will focus on the earlier techniques.)

Now consider what might happen if, in the 1980s, the model Claudia Schiffer and the professional skier Picabo Street were skiing together and each tore an ACL. Hearing the same information about the options available, the two would likely choose differently. Ms. Street would likely choose the strength-restoring surgery that comes with large scars; Ms. Schiffer would likely choose lower knee function with smaller scars. By allowing each to continue in her chosen profession, these choices would be best for the women's health qua persons. Would Ms. Schiffer's choice really be worse for her qua organism? It might seem so, because she is left with reduced functioning. On the other hand, her appearance earns her a great deal of money and maintains her social network, so more biological goals might be served by her not taking the steps necessary to restore function in her knee. Whereas a person who simply does not desire to eat, or who chooses to smoke tobacco with full knowledge of its effects, can present a true conflict between health qua person and health qua organism, these examples illustrate how very unclear the boundary between the two sides can be.

Due to lack of insight that can accompany illness, it may be difficult to distinguish between an addiction and a goal. Someone who reports a constant desire for whiskey may have an alcohol addiction or may just have a goal that is in conflict with his health as an organism. In this section we are primarily interested in the latter case. As for the former, it might be appropriate to describe the alcoholic's desire for a drink not as a goal so much as an appetite. His goal is better described as quelling the appetite or as not having that appetite rule his actions. A better example of a person for whom health qua person conflicts with health qua organism is this individual who is not an alcoholic but who simply desires to drink large quantities of alcohol often. No doubt many American college students fall into this category. Other examples include the man who wants a vasectomy and the woman who wants to take birth control pills.

Often individuals act in ways that threaten to sacrifice their health qua organisms without conscious consideration. However, in other cases the choice is made with clear deliberation, as it was when Witty Ticcy Ray decided to refrain from taking his medication in order to improve his musical performances, or when an intelligent adult without addiction chooses to go on a drinking binge. Another case is the philosopher or physician who chooses to contract a deadly disease in order to understand what this experience is like, or the Indian woman who desires to perform suttee, ritual suicide on the funeral pyre of her dead husband. We can stipulate that these goals are real, stable constituents of a coherent set of goals embraced by informed individuals. They are not to be rejected on the basis that they are not really part of what determines the health of the individuals qua persons. We have noted that duties, specifically duties of medical beneficence, can conflict with other duties. What we have here are conflicting duties of medical beneficence.

But these cases do not all seem the same. The more serious the impact or risk to the health of the individual qua organism, the more we have the sense that it must be impermissible to pursue health qua person. Why is that? Are not persons more important than mere organisms? A principle of beneficence cannot help us determine an HCP's actual duty when the prima facie duty to improve the health of the patient qua person conflicts with the prima facie duty to improve the health of the patient qua organism. For this we need an account of the force and limits of the duty to respect the choices of individuals. That is, we have to consider the character of autonomy. This is the focus of the next chapter.

Postscript: Enhancement

The proliferation of new medical technologies has drawn attention to the ways in which interventions can be applied to improve individuals beyond what is usually considered healthy and into what Boorse (1977) and others called "positive health." One result is a distinction between treatment (therapy) and enhancement.

Buchanan et al. (2000, 110) distinguished between, on the one hand, ". . . services or interventions meant to prevent or cure (or otherwise ameliorate) conditions viewed as diseases or impairments . . .", and, on the other hand, ". . . interventions that improve a condition viewed as a normal function or features of members of our species." The first is treatment, the second enhancement. These authors linked the idea of enhancement to the concept of "medical necessity" that is used to determine what health insurance will cover. The idea is that bringing people to health is medically necessary, but super-health from enhancement is not.

Francis Fukuyama (2002) saw the controversial emergence of ADHD diagnoses and treatment with Ritalin as a classic example of society grappling with the distinction between therapy and enhancement. Many still have a sense that Ritalin is prescribed more to push individuals into positive health (enhancement) than to treat a disease (therapy). This sense has been fading as the public accepts ADHD as unhealthy. The distinction between therapy and enhancement is also central to the issue of doping in sports. Fukuyama is partially responsible for promoting the terms "posthuman" and "posthumanism" to describe efforts to enhance people beyond what has been considered normal and healthy.

What sense can we make of the treatment-enhancement distinction in the context of the Richman–Budson theory of health? We might take enhancement to involve raising both abilities and goals of individuals qua organisms. This would make enhancement of organisms parallel to quality of life of persons. Raising an organism's goals and abilities in tandem maintains the organism's level of health, but somehow enriches the organism. It would be reasonable to understand enhancement in this way. (Whether it is possible to raise biological goals is another matter, and one that will not be settled here.)

If we hold biological goals as given, enhancement becomes intentional increase in abilities beyond what is usually available for reaching standard goals. Obviously, this gloss contains a promissory note for explanations of 'usually' and 'standard.'

An intervention counts as enhancement only if the individual is already healthy, at least with respect to the area in which abilities are being enhanced. This means that enhancement cannot be what makes an individual healthy. What if an intervention raises both biological goals and biological abilities beyond what is standard, but leaves the abilities falling short of the goals? We may find ourselves calling this enhancement even though the individual technically speaking is less healthy qua organism. Interventions that increase abilities in ways unconnected to biological function do not count as enhancement in the sense we are interested in here. Such interventions would more rightly be called self-improvement, education, or skill building.

Enhancement involves tweaking the biological bases of our abilities. However, whether we count a given intervention as enhancement may depend on whether we are thinking of the individual qua organism or qua person. Consider a person who is healthy qua organism but unhealthy qua person. Improving biological function in a way that makes him healthier qua person would count as enhancement for the individual qua organism, but as health care and not enhancement for the individual qua person.

Enhancement raises the same ethical issues as quality of life, plus additional ones to boot. In the framework I have been developing, enhancement as such does not fall under a duty of medical beneficence because it does not improve the health of individuals. Insofar as it can improve people's lives, it may fall under a more general duty of beneficence in the same way that improving quality of life does. At the same time, insofar as enhancement is characteristically pursued using the tools of medicine, this aspect of the general duty of beneficence may fall primarily to HCPs.

Many worries have been raised about the permissibility of beneficence through enhancement, including justice and equal opportunity and respect for the natural. Such weighty issues must indeed be taken into account in applying medical techniques to those who are already healthy. Once again, I plead immunity, as these important issues fall outside the scope of the current project.

4

Autonomy and Parentalism

Chapter 3 identified a duty of medical beneficence, being a duty of health care professionals (HCPs) to improve the health of an individual. I distinguished this duty from the related duty to improve patients' quality of life. At the end of chapter 3 we found that in cases in which improving the health of the patient qua person requires lowering the health of the patient qua organism, HCPs face conflicting duties of medical beneficence. To address this conflict, we now turn to the topic of autonomy. In this chapter I propose that we have reason to respect the goals of persons and to prefer satisfying these goals to satisfying the goals of the same individuals qua organisms.

I began the last chapter by emphasizing that the Richman–Budson theory is a theory of health, so that HCPs have to collect data on patients' personal goals in order to determine what will improve patients' health qua persons. This is a metaphysical claim that helps us to understand how the duty of medical beneficence is fulfilled. But patients' goals are not only central to determining what will make them healthy, they are also key to patient autonomy. Thus, the duty to respect patient autonomy coheres explicitly with our metaphysical account of health of individuals qua persons. Furthermore, if we take health of persons to be determined by the goals of persons, beneficence and autonomy, often understood to be at odds, actually converge. I take the (mutual) coherence of these metaphysical and ethical theses to be support for both.

Remarks on Ethics: Duties and Goods

I have stated that health is a good. It has intrinsic value and (which is not the same thing) is one of the things that we want. Our actions should seek to maximize health. Health is not the only good, however; others include happiness, justice, autonomy, and perhaps even beauty, and our actions should also seek to maximize them. Obviously, we cannot maximize all goods all the time. Although this book is not about goods other than health, we must recognize the necessity of trade-offs between health and other goods.

In talking about competing goods, it is helpful to return to the distinction between a prima facie duty and an actual duty, mentioned in the previous chapter. The intrinsic value of happiness may make it our duty to maximize the total amount of happiness in the world, but doing this may conflict with our duty to distribute goods justly. Following W. D. Ross, we might say that, in such a situation, both courses of action can be called prima facie duties, but only one can be our *actual* duty. Actions that are prima facie duties are obligatory unless, in a given situation, an overriding stronger (or perhaps equal) obligation conflicts with it. One's actual duty is determined by considering all of the prima facie duties and their relative weights (strengths). "What agents ought to do is, in the end, determined by what they ought to do *all things considered*" (Beauchamp and Childress 2001, 15). Whereas we must eventually determine our actual duty, identifying our prima facie obligations is itself a project.

We might begin to specify these obligations by adopting principles. Bioethicists using this approach, often called *principlism*, generally identify four principles as the guiding prima facie duties relevant to health care. They come in a variety of formulations, but can be represented as follows:

Principle of beneficence: HCPs have a duty to benefit patients.

Principle of nonmaleficence: HCPs have a duty not to harm patients.

Principle of autonomy: HCPs have a duty not to interfere with the right of patients to choose what happens to themselves.

Principle of justice: Goods should be distributed fairly.

Ronald Munson's book *Intervention and Reflection*, one of the most widely used medical ethics textbooks, introduces medical ethics with heavy emphasis on principles (Munson 2000, 30–45). Beauchamp and Childress (2001, 23) identified themselves as principlists. Engelhardt (1996, chapter 3) also relied heavily on principles.

Apposite to principlism is *casuistry*. As a method, casuistry starts with assessment of particular cases, supporting conclusions about new and more ambiguous cases by drawing analogies to ones for which the moral status is more clear.

Casuists often take principlists to task for failing to prove the authority of the principles and for inappropriately applying intellectual, a priori conclusions to real life cases:

> As a dialectical method of moral reasoning inspired by Aristotle and Aquinas, casuistry may well prove relevant . . . in virtue of its opposition to inflexible and literal interpretations of moral principles, and its resistance to any ethical attitude which first absolutizes a universal moral norm and then insists on its all-round and unyielding application, while denying any abatement or adjustment to changing contingencies. (Stone 1998, 228)

Having roots in real cases, in the same type of material to which its conclusions will be applied, makes casuistry seem well grounded. Its similarity to the case method in law makes it seem familiar.

However, casuistry is vulnerable to attacks on the authority of our judgment of particular cases and on the validity of analogical reasoning. It is also vulnerable to the objection that it draws normative conclusions from factual premises. Principlists at least know what makes the inference to a normative conclusion *logically* valid—we introduce an ought (I used "duty" in my formulations above) when we make a principle a premise of our reasoning.

In practice, the contrast between casuistry and principlism ends up looking like one of emphasis. Consider Jonsen and Toulmin's description of casuistry as:

> . . . the analysis of moral issues, using procedures of reasoning based on paradigms and analogies, leading to the formulation of expert opinion about the existence and stringency of particular moral obligations, framed in terms of rules and maxims that are general but not universal or invariable, since they hold good with certainty only in the typical conditions of the agent and circumstances of the case. (Jonsen and Toulmin 1988, 257, quoted in Jonsen 1995, 348)

Casuists start with particular cases, drawing analogies between paradigm cases and these under scrutiny; principlists start with universal principles. Neither method is pure and neither stands alone. Casuistry is too inefficient without general rules and maxims; principles that fail to fit our assessment of particular cases lose their authority.

I endorse a hybrid approach, which Beauchamp and Childress (2001, 397ff) call "coherentism." Principles are checked against cases and amended appropriately, and assessment of duty in particular cases is checked against principles in a process John Rawls (1971) called "reflective equilibrium." What we want out of this process is precisely what we want when we assess theories in any other domain. We want a theory that exhibits those features we value in theories: covering and explaining the data, simplicity, and so on. And, as in other domains, we will sometimes reinterpret particular cases according to the theory we are trying out.

I intend this approach to ethics to be consistent with my approach to the formulation of a theory of health. In part I of this book we considered theories of health by examining them for internal coherence and theoretical plausibility, and by checking them against cases. Our initial considerations were theoretical. When the theoretical seemed to clash with intuitions concerning particular cases, we considered adjusting the theory. For instance, after considering individuals with goals that are self-defeating in ways that such individuals could not be expected to appreciate, I amended the theory by introducing the notion of an ideal observer. We also allowed reconsideration of intuitions, as after examining the case of Witty Ticcy Ray's weekend plans.

In ethics, as in metaphysics, the data underdetermine theory. In other words, the same data will be consistent with any number of different explanations. (Quine, Duhem, and others made this point forcefully and famously.) Consider also that our theory about an area of inquiry helps form our understanding of the very content of this area of inquiry. Kuhn (1962) is famous for making this point. (See also McMullin 1995.) This gives us reasons for starting with theory rather than with raw data. This is especially true if we have independent support for a theory. I believe we may have such support for a principle of autonomy. In the following sections we will examine some of that support.

Autonomy is at issue because we have to sort out what to do in the face of the conflicts discussed at the end of the last chapter. There we saw that appealing to the HCP's duty of medical beneficence will not help us when efforts to improve the patient's health qua person are in conflict with the patient's health qua organism. We need another tool, one that identifies an actual duty in the face of conflicting prima facie duties, one that will explain the force and limits of the respect for persons driving our intuition that health qua person trumps health qua organism. This tool is autonomy.

Autonomy: The Big Idea

A principle of autonomy can be formulated in several ways. Ethicists have described autonomy variously in terms of the HCP's duty to respect patients' wishes, as patients' right to self-determination, or even as a duty of patients to make decisions when they are capable of doing so. The capacity for autonomy and the bearers of this capacity have also been treated as inherently valuable. The big idea is that, ceteris paribus, what an individual wants for his or her own life carries more weight than does what others want for his or her life.

For their account of autonomy, Beauchamp and Childress (2001, 59) take as central the idea of *autonomous action*. They "... analyze autonomous action in terms of normal choosers who act (1) intentionally, (2) with understanding, and (3) without controlling influences that determine their action."[1] Each of these conditions is important as a sign that the chooser is the agent rather than an object of the action in question. Autonomous action bears an authority that obligates HCPs:

Respect for autonomy is not a mere *ideal* in health care; it is a professional *obligation*. Autonomous choice is a *right*, not a *duty* of patients. (Beauchamp and Childress 2001, 63)

The big idea: when a patient makes an autonomous choice, HCPs are obligated to respect that choice.

Beauchamp and Childress's analysis allows that autonomous action is subject to failure on four planes: failure of the chooser to be normal, failure of intention, failure of understanding, and failure of freedom from controlling influences. Any given action is likely to face some limitation on at least one of these. (Beauchamp and Childress claim that, unlike the other criteria, whether an action is intentional is not a matter of degree, but this may not be obvious.) Indeed, this is especially true of actions by those in ill health. Aware of this, those authors do not demand that an action comply strictly with their criteria in order to deserve respect from HCPs.[2] In their view, to retain respect for autonomous action as an actual (or as actually a prima facie) obligation of HCPs, we must apply the concept of autonomous action in a way such that many actual actions count as autonomous "enough."

Engelhardt captured respect for autonomy under what he named the principle of permission. This principle states, "Authority for actions involving others in a secular pluralist society is derived from their permission" (Engelhardt 1996, 122). This approach arises out of Engelhardt's thesis that in communities that are not governed by a single religion-based ethical code and that embrace diversity (such as many take the American ideal to be), the authority of moral claims comes from agreement (Engelhardt 1996, 67ff). That is, an action that will affect me or, as in the case of medical treatment, that is intended to benefit me, is permissible only if I agree that it is permissible. The principle of permission provides a maxim for guiding actions: "Do not do to others that which they would not have done unto them, and do for them that which one has contracted to do" (Engelhardt 1996, 123).

Aside from administration (e.g., billing, supervision of staff) and education (e.g., supervising students, answering patients' questions), the primary activities of medical personnel are treatment and research. These are distinguished by their purposes. The purpose of medical treatment (therapy) is to benefit the patient; the purpose of research is to increase knowledge. (Research subjects may hope to benefit from their participation, but such benefit is not characteristic of research as such.) Permission and respect for autonomy are of obvious importance for research. The big idea is that respect for autonomy is important even in therapeutic interactions—that is, even when we are attempting to fulfill a duty of medical beneficence.

Autonomy—A Kantian Exposition

I suggested above that there is independent theoretical support for a principle of autonomy. This section presents autonomy as a theoretical concept. Although bioethicists such as Beauchamp and Childress treat autonomy as the subject of its own principle, the Belmont Report (the document that shaped American views on the ethics of research involving human subjects) includes respect for autonomy under a more general principle of respect for persons. That includes protection of vulnerable populations, those whose capacities for making free and rational decisions are compromised by institutionalization, age, mental deficits, social status, or other factors. Including autonomy under the rubric of respect for persons highlights the idea that autonomy is an important part of our view of what it is to be a person. As I noted in chapter 2, this way of thinking about autonomy found its most elegant and weighty formulation in Kant's systematic ethical theory. The role of autonomy in such a coherent system provides the kind of theoretical support for a principle of autonomy that we are looking for.

In this section, I offer a Kantian account of autonomy. I do not claim completeness or sensitivity to the nuances of Kant's texts or historical context. I hope only to show something of the strength and beauty of his approach.

Central to a Kantian theory of ethics is the doctrine that human beings have intrinsic value. This is captured in the second formulation of the categorical imperative, which enjoins us to *treat humanity, whether in ourselves or in others, always as an end in itself and never only as a means* (Kant 1959, 47). Treating a woman as an end in herself is treating her as intrinsically valuable; treating her as a means is treating her as having instrumental value. Thus, Kant does not prohibit treating individuals as means to some other end as long as they are also being treated as ends in themselves:

Now, I say, man and, in general, every rational being exists as an end in himself and not merely as a means to be arbitrarily used by this or that will. In all his actions, whether they are directed to himself or to other rational beings, he must always be regarded at the same time as an end. (Kant 1959, 46)

Commentators have given different names to this imperative; for example, the "Formula of the End-in-Itself" (O'Neill 1989, 341). I call it the principle of dignity, as it specifies an obligation to respect each rational being as having inherent worth.

We are ends in ourselves precisely because we have within ourselves the source of moral obligation: "A rational being belongs to the realm of ends as a member when he gives universal laws in it while also himself subject to these laws" (Kant 1959, 52). We have impulses and desires, motivations, goals, and interests. In deciding how to act on these, we engage reason, the distinctively human faculty. The central characteristic of reason is the function of drawing connections among similar items—the ability to universalize, to consider a possible action as an instance of a *law* for action. A rational creature understands that it is permissible to act on a particular motive in the present situation only if it is permissible to act on that motive in every situation that is relevantly similar. That is, a rational creature understands that if any of the relevantly similar situations are such that it is not permissible to act on that motive, it could not be permissible to act on that motive in the present situation. Given the assumption that all human beings are at core the same, we see that the fact that an action is being done by someone else rather than by oneself does not by itself constitute a relevant difference.

Thus, when considering whether to act on a particular motive in a particular situation, the Kantian thinks about whether the motive, the "maxim" of the action, can be applied universally. The first of Kant's formulations of the categorical imperative captures this: *act only in such a way that you could will the maxim of your action to be a universal law* (cf. Kant 1959, 39). O'Neill called this formulation of the categorical imperative the formula of universal law. I call it the principle of universalizability because it indicates that no maxim is a permissible one unless it can be made universal.[3] The capacity, indeed the need, for motivations and maxims (reasons for action) is part of our humanity. So is rationality—the faculty of seeing a universal—that allows us to recognize when a maxim is a particular instance of a possible law. The universalized versions of bad maxims are impossible in the sense that they are self-contradictory and cannot be put into universal practice.

When we exercise our rationality and embrace those of our maxims that are universalizable, we give ourselves laws. Thus, our experience as rational agents is one of literal auto-nomy. Acting on laws is acting consistently and from reasons. As the source of laws, we are, as Kant put it, sovereign beings. It is our very status as the source of moral law that makes us members of the "kingdom of ends," a kingdom in which all are sovereign and all have intrinsic value.

Kant connected this account of autonomy with a broader theory of causation. To count as having been caused at all, an event must follow from its cause according to a law. Where no law connects two events, we cannot call one the cause of the other. Thus in order for us to be the causes of our own actions, these actions must conform to laws.

It is sometimes jarring when we realize that to be truly free (autonomous) involves acting in consistent and hence predictable ways. We tend to think of free action as spontaneous in the sense of unpredictable. However, the idea that freedom is not the same as simple spontaneity or unpredictability has a long history (in Spinoza, Leibniz, Hume, et al.). It is also well rooted in the practice of clinical ethics, where it is common to assess whether a patient's choice is autonomous by determining whether it is consistent with his or her previous choices.

Cassell (1997, 17) contrasted two cases to show how this can be applied:

When the man with meningitis refuses treatment and asks to be allowed to die, it does not appear to me to be a truly autonomous act. However, when a dialysand refuses further dialysis, his action appear[s] to me to be much more the exercise of his autonomy.

The dialysand has established a relationship with the medical staff over a period of regular treatments. His HCPs are thus in a position to judge whether the decision to refuse further treatment is consistent with his other choices and values. When we judge whether a decision has been made autonomously by looking for patterns in a patient's choices, we are applying a Kantian notion of autonomy. We are looking to see whether the patient is acting according to a principle of universalizability.

On the Impossibility of Autonomy

With or without that Kantian analysis, the idea that patient autonomy should play a central role in determining how medical care is provided is subject to some very powerful objections. Some will be familiar as objections to "liberal" political theory; others are specific to the medical context. In this section I sketch some of these objections, divided into those based on rejection of values associated with autonomy, on irrationality, on rejection of the individual, on the nature of the role of patient, on the claim that many patients do not want autonomy, and on improper application of the concept. Each of these could be a chapter of a book on autonomy; here I will only sketch each type. In the next section I will attempt to pick up the pieces and show that, despite real limitations, respect for autonomy is still possible and obligatory in medical encounters both common and extreme.

Objections Based on Rejection of Associated Values

The first and last types of objections are unlike the others we will consider in that they do not give reasons for thinking that autonomy is impossible. Instead, they raise questions about whether the concept gets us what we want. Objections of the first type suggest that the emphasis on autonomy that has developed in ethics and politics has been supported by and has fostered a questionable set of values. A feminist critique of the "symbolic meaning" of the autonomous individual rejects the "cultural character ideal" that naïve adherence to a theory of autonomy fosters. Whereas a feminist ethics of care emphasizes community, interconnectedness, and relationships, an ethic based on autonomy emphasizes individuals and ". . . promotes a very stripped-down conception of agents as atomistic bearers of rights, a conception in which the diversity and complexity of agents are pared away and agents are reduced to an interchangeable sameness" (Mackenzie and Stoljar 2000, 6).

According to this critique, putting autonomy at the center means pushing relationships and mutuality aside, and that means putting women aside:

... traditional conceptions of autonomy not only disvalue women's experience and those values arising from it, such as love, loyalty, friendship, and care, but also are defined in opposition to femininity. Traditional conceptions are thus masculinist conceptions. (Mackenzie and Stoljar 2000, 9)

One point of this critique is that the moral agent is understood as autonomous in the traditional sense (as independent, atomistic, and rational) only at the cost of excluding women from the class of moral agents, and this is too high a cost. Identification of alternative values with women is supported by both theoretical arguments (Code 2000) and empirical studies (Gilligan 1982).

Objections Based on Irrationality of Persons

This objection cites the fact that human beings simply are not rational. According to several studies (Nisbett and Ross 1980; Tversky and Kahneman 1982; Wason and Johnson-Laird 1972), we are consistently and predictably bad at a variety of reasoning tasks.[4] Many of the mistakes studied involve fallacious inferences about probabilities (e.g., the gambler's fallacy[5]). Others involve bad reasoning about reasoning, in which subjects give wrong answers to questions about what further information would be relevant for drawing conclusions from a given set of data. In philosophy, some of the best-known discussions of this literature are by Stephen Stich (1990, 1981).[6]

The significance of these findings for us is that if we must be rational in order to be autonomous, then autonomy should not be expected and thus cannot be used to identify binding obligations. This follows with the help of the principle that "ought implies can." We are never obligated to do something that we are simply unable to do.

Objections Based on Rejection of the Individual

Traditional ways of thinking about autonomy also come under fire from those who reject as false the notion that we are individuals who deliberate and make rational choices about our lives. One theory, for instance, posits that persons are not just influenced but are in part *constituted* by their relationships:

Being in relationships is ontologically significant in the sense that it is the background against which content is given to that which is of fundamental value to liberals, an individual's freedom to plan and manage a life. In relationships with others in a community of relationships content is given to such basic human capacities as pursuing, questioning, exploring, developing, and actualizing interests, projects, and goals. (Koggel 1998, 143)

In this picture, the idea of an autonomous individual person is incoherent because our very personhood depends on others.[7] There is nothing in the world to which the label "autonomous individual" applies. Other arguments against the traditional idea of an individual can be generated from Freudian views of the self as made up of several forces that are often at odds, from Foucauldian analyses of agency,[8] and from tenets of identity politics and multiculturalism.[9]

Communitarian critiques of atomism seem to waver between two reasons for adopting a social conception of the self: because such a conception provides a more accurate reflection of what selves are really like, and because, independent of ontological issues, it produces better ethics and politics. In the view of Linda L. and Ezekiel J. Emanuel (1993), autonomy should be understood in terms of community preferences, not just individual ones. For the communitarian, the ethical unit is the community rather than the individual.

Objections Based on the Nature of the Role of the Patient

Another line of reasoning explains that autonomy is not a concept that applies to individuals in the role of patients. After all, the very idea of a patient is of someone who is passive, the recipient of care rather than the agent of care.[10] Autonomy applies to agents: those who are active and acting. To apply the concept of autonomy to a patient seems like a category mistake.

Even were we to maintain that those seeking medical care should not be called "patients" or put in the role of a passive recipient, it is still the case that agency is diminished by illness. Recall the claim that illness affects each of four features of autonomy: "self-direction, establishing a life plan, deliberating about applying a life plan (reasoning and information), and acting on the basis of such deliberations" (Pellegrino and Thomasma 1988, 17). Being unwell typically involves (or is even constituted by) diminution of our abilities of self-direction, deliberation, and action. It would thus seem that the demand to respect patient autonomy fails to connect with the patient's reality. The times when we are most in need of medical care are those when we are least able to be autonomous.

Objections Based on the Claim That Many Patients Do Not Want Autonomy

Some question the desire of patients to exercise autonomy when it comes to their medical care. Carl E. Schneider (1998, 75) wrote, "The autonomy paradigm rests on assumptions about the natural desire of all people to control themselves and their surroundings . . . I . . . contend . . . [that] these assumptions are overstated even for the population at large." To sum up Schneider's conclusion, ". . . to make autonomy a mandatory duty of patients, as some bioethicists imply, would seem to be an unrealistic moral imposition and a violation of autonomy, itself" (Pellegrino 2000, 362). The ideal of the autonomous patient makes sense in application only if patients *want* to make their own decisions. If, as Schneider suggested, patients often want to exercise the freedom to have someone else choose, we may be able to do little in response.

Objections Based on Improper Application

In the context of clinical bioethics, autonomy is closely linked with competence and informed consent. Patients who are not competent cannot exercise autonomy; those who cannot exercise autonomy cannot give informed consent to treatment or informed refusal of treatment. "When patients are judged incompetent, they forfeit their autonomy to decide about their medical care, the power to do so being transferred to others who will exercise it on patients' behalf" (Grisso and Appelbaum 1998, 148). Where individual autonomy is held as a central value, as it is in the United States and other Western democracies, HCPs may not treat competent patients without their consent. However, if a patient is deemed incompetent, decisions for care are appropriately made by others.

The final objection that we review here is based on the claim that the ideal of autonomy is often invoked in order to have a patient declared incompetent when what is really going on is that the patient's HCPs or family members do not want to comply with the patient's requests. It is easy to see how HCPs and interested parties who cannot understand or who disagree with the values driving a patient's decision can come to the conclusion that the patient is irrational and hence not autonomous. This conclusion is often used to support a decision to treat a patient against his or her will. The flip side of this is that HCPs can use "respecting patient autonomy" as an excuse to *abandon* those who need treatment and are resistant due to fear, misunderstanding, or incapacity. The fact that autonomy has been abused in these ways makes some bioethicists wary of allowing it to play an important role in clinical ethics.

Reconstructing Autonomy

Although these issues are very real, I believe that an important and useful conception of autonomy can yet survive. In this section I suggest looking to the concept of a *practical identity* to reframe our understanding of autonomy in a way that better reflects real values and real people. We will see that many misuses of the traditional view of autonomy occur because we are looking at decisions on the wrong level. We do not commonly form maxims and goals having to do with specific medical procedures. Rather, our life plans and self-conceptions are formed along lines both more general ("I am a teacher") and more specific ("I value being able to hug my wife").

Korsgaard on Practical Identities

Philosopher Christine Korsgaard developed an approach to ethics that emphasizes the particular motivations and identities of individuals while remaining grounded in Kant's theory of a universal rational human nature. She understood Kantian ethics to provide an account of value that answers to the intuitions of both the realist and the empiricist about moral values, much as embedded instrumentalist accounts of health answer to the intuitions that health is objective and the same for all, and yet at some level subjective and quite idiosyncratic for each person. Reworking Kant's concept of a hypothetical imperative, Korsgaard proposed that there is value in satisfying the autonomous choices of rational agents:

The *objects* of value are just the things that are important to us, the objects of natural human interests. But the resulting values are not "subjective" or given directly by those interests. Value springs from the act of rational choice. Our commitment to the value of humanity constrains our own choices, by limiting us to pursuits which are acceptable from the standpoint of others, and extending our concern to the things which others choose. . . . What brings "objectivity" to the realm of values is not that certain things *have* objective value, but rather that there are constraints on rational choice. (Korsgaard 1996a, x)

Korsgaard's Kantian ethics tells us that to find out how to fulfill our obligations we must collect contingent facts about what real people actually want. These actual wants have objective value insofar as they follow from or conform to the humanity of those who adopt them; that is, insofar as they conform to constraints of rationality (universalizability).[11]

As our rationality is what makes us members of the kingdom of ends, it is only when we exercise it that our will (which is itself, for Kant, practical *reason*[12]) determines ends in a way that confers objective value. For Korsgaard, the practical reason of individuals can confer value even on ends that would otherwise not bind others. For her, this is an aspect of the principle of dignity (*treat humanity, whether in yourself or in others, as an end in itself and never as a means only*), which she called the "formula of humanity":

. . . it is the capacity for the rational determination of ends in general, not just the capacity for adopting morally obligatory ends, that the Formula of Humanity orders us to cherish unconditionally. (Korsgaard 1996a, 111)

Morally obligatory ends are ends that bind the actions of all rational beings independent of any contingent interests or identities. But our humanity enables us to choose other ends as well. When an end is chosen "under the influence of reason," ". . . it is to be deemed important or valuable, not because it contributes to survival or instinctual satisfaction, but as an end—for its own sake" (Korsgaard 1996a, 114).[13]

These contingent ends arise from our "practical identities." A practical identity is ". . . a description under which you value yourself, a description under which you find your life to be worth living and your actions to be worth undertaking" (Korsgaard 1996b, 101).

Practical identity is a complex matter and for the average person there will be a jumble of such conceptions. You are a human being, a woman or a man, an adherent of a certain religion, a member of an ethnic group, a member of a certain profession, someone's lover or friend, and so on. And all of these identities give rise to reasons and obligations. (Korsgaard 1996b, 101)

Our practical identities are sometimes what we choose purposefully and sometimes simply the result of accidents of upbringing or experience.[14] Even so, in adopting them we adopt ends, reasons for acting. In embracing my identity as an American citizen, I make the welfare of my country an end for me; in embracing my identity as Matt's teacher, I make Matt's education an end for me.[15]

But in what way do the ends I choose bear on the obligations of others? What gives these subjective values objectivity (in the sense of intersubjectivity)? The lawlike character of my own reasons does:

> The reflective structure of human consciousness requires that you identify yourself with some law or principle which will govern your choices. It requires you to be a law to yourself. And that is the source of normativity. (Korsgaard 1996b, 103–04)

The required universalizability of our rational choices is what makes our own reasons for others, as well.

If someone is treating me ill, I can obligate him to stop by appealing to the fact that universalizing his action would be unacceptable. I do this by saying, *How would you like it if someone did that to you?* (Korsgaard 1996b, 142). After hearing this, the other person is given a reason, even an obligation, to cease the objectionable behavior. This obligation is grounded in the status of the other as an end in herself. "But if you are a law to others in so far as you are just human, just *someone*, then the humanity of others is also a law to you" (Korsgaard 1996b, 143). The appeal to consistency just makes explicit the universalizability requirement; the reason is only a reason for me if it is also a reason for you.

My practical identities bind others because others recognize that they would be bound by them if they adopted the same identities. We also recognize that acting according to maxims that issue from practical identities is part of what makes someone a member of the kingdom of ends. It would not make sense to interpret this as meaning that "... it does not ... matter whose end an end is" (Herman 1984, 600). For surely I am not obligated to pursue your ends as diligently as my own. Rather:

> What I support is the other's active and successful pursuit of his self-defined goals. ... That is, what I have a duty to do is to contribute to the meeting of his true needs when that is not within his power. ... ... in taking another's ends as my own, or his happiness as an obligatory end, I acknowledge him as a member of the community of mutual aid. (Herman 1984, 600)

Respecting another as an end requires supporting the person as one who pursues the ends of his or her own choosing.

Some will object that autonomy in this mode will be impossible more often than not because our self-conceptions are always shifting. Due to declining membership in religious and service organizations and changes in structure of careers and the workplace, this objection carries more weight now than it would have 100 or even 50 years ago. It is true that individuals are, in general, less likely than in earlier times to think of their involvement with the Boy Scouts of America, the Benevolent and Protective Order of Elks, or the Junior League as determining a practical identity for them and as contributing to how they should behave. Our working lives have also changed. With the decline of guilds and unions, people identify much less with their professions than they used to. Not so long ago it was possible to stand on certain street corners in Philadelphia or London and tell with a fair degree of certainty whether the man passing by was a lawyer, banker, or architect without having to be a Sherlock Holmes or a John Steed. No longer.

Despite these trends, people still hold onto practical identities in myriad public and private ways, and expect others to act in ways appropriate to theirs. The importance of these identities is reflected in the journalistic practice of adding identity ascriptions to names, so that individuals are referred to with phrases such as "American artist Jackson Pollack," and "folk singer Arlo Guthrie, son of Woody Guthrie." Practical identities are also used to express judgments about the behavior of others. We say, "How could a mother do such a thing," or "And he calls himself a veterinarian!" My professional identity has seemed perfectly obvious to at least several strangers. One morning in Kalamazoo, while waiting for the oil to be changed in my car, I was approached by a student from a nearby university where I had never taught or even lectured. With only the introduction, "You're a philosophy professor, right?", she launched into a series of questions about Leibniz![16]

Do Constraints of Reason Constrain Health-Determining Goals?

I have claimed that a state of health, being a sort of equilibrium between our abilities and our goals, is intrinsically valuable. Since the goals of individuals vary and the states to which they refer or that could serve to fulfill them do not carry value themselves, these goals have instrumental value that can be thought of as "embedded" in the intrinsic value of the healthy state that they in part determine. In developing what might be called my philosophy of medicine, I adopted a Kantian view according to which, what makes the pursuit of goals valuable is that they are the goals of autonomous individuals. I follow Christine Korsgaard in thinking that the goals of autonomous individuals give us reasons for action, and in conceiving of goals as falling into clusters around people's practical identities. This allows us to explain why it is that the health of a patient qua person is to be respected over the health of the same patient qua organism, allows us to make sense of autonomy in imperfectly rational individuals, and shows how we may assess whether a given treatment supports a patient's autonomy even when that patient cannot provide explicit consent. Much of this benefit is explicated in what follows.

Korsgaard proposed that only intentions conforming to the limits of reason give us reasons.[17] This is consistent with Kant's view that morally wrong actions are not truly autonomous. We rehearsed the reasoning behind this view, starting with the idea that autonomy is giving oneself laws for action, adopting the maxims of one's actions as universal rules for action in general. Add to this the thesis, corollary to the first formulation of the categorical imperative, that attempts to universalize immoral maxims yield contradictions, and we have the result that immoral goals do not warrant respect because they are not true examples of autonomy. Linking autonomy, rationality, and permissibility in this way suggests that a process of goal clarification (increasing the rationality of one's set of practical identities and goals) would also be a process in which immoral goals would be eliminated.

Does this mean that bad people cannot be autonomous? Although I am drawn to the idea that immoral choices tend to be irrational choices, it also seems more than likely that some individuals embrace goals—even whole practical identities—that are immoral. No doubt, curtain card sharks, rat finks, cat burglars, and pimps willingly, even thoughtfully, embrace these identities. (Think of Tony Soprano, the television character who continues to embrace his identity as a gangster even while in psychotherapy.) Even if a Kantian would be correct to suggest that these identities violate the bounds of rationality very strictly understood, we must allow that people do adopt such goals. Otherwise, we are caught with a notion bearing little relation to actual human beings. In addition, I want to hold onto a distinction between health and ethics. A strict application of the notion that goals are autonomous and confer value only when strictly rational, combined with the thesis that rationality is the test of permissibility, would make the range of permissible goals coextensive with the range of goals relevant to assessment of health status.

In short, I want to hold (with the Kantian) that autonomous choices of individuals confer value, and also hold (with the Humean) that no desire is by itself contrary to reason. This is not to say that an individual's goals cannot be contradictory or self-defeating. Chapter 2 describes several ways in which an individual's goals can be sufficiently problematic as to fail to form a coherent set that can serve to frame what would count as healthy for that individual qua person. Immoral goals need not have incoherencies of that order. Immoral sets of goals (including those of Mr. Sloth) that do not suffer from the incoherencies identified in chapter 2 can determine what counts as health for individuals qua persons. As noted, where patients have such goals, the HCP may face a conflict between ethical duties and medical duties.

Practical Identities in the Medical Context

Since we establish rules for ourselves on the basis of practical identities, it is on this basis that we must understand the exercise of and respect for autonomy. We can adopt these identities even when we cannot realize them without help, and even when we do not even know what will help us to realize them.[18] The constraints of other ethical principles allow us to withhold respect for certain identities. For Korsgaard and other Kantians, unacceptable identities such as those of a liar, a thief, and a murderer, generally lie outside the constraints of rationality.

Understanding autonomy in terms of practical identities helps us to see ways in which the medical context poses real challenges. One way is that illness causes people to reevaluate their identities: ". . . the suddenness and significance of some healthcare crises force a radical reassessment of one's self-understanding, which may effectively derail a person's autonomy competency" (Dodds 2000, 230). We cannot be autonomous except when we have rules for decision making, and we make such rules in part as they relate to our practical identities. However, many health care decisions must be made when our practical identities are under fire. A calligrapher who has lost her hands in an industrial accident will have to adjust her practical identities, and until she does so in a settled way she may face some decisions for which she is unable to draw upon a rule or identity that can serve as the basis of autonomous choice. Where the patient's practical identities are really up in the air, it is certainly best to maximize health qua organism. This is because a healthy organism is most likely to support health of the patient qua person whatever the patient's practical identities turn out to be once they are more stable.

It is well known that an identity as a devout Roman Catholic, for example, comes with certain medical imperatives (albeit ones that many opt out of), but what about an identity as a mathematician or a dancer? Maxims that accompany most practical identities can be specified in terms of valued abilities or preferences among activities. As I noted above, compared with questions of whether to choose a particular medication or therapeutic procedure, such maxims can be at a very high level of generality. I am David's son, but this does not by itself make me a person who chooses surgery over drug therapy or relief from pain over mental alertness.

With the exception of those who adopt practical identities as members of disability communities or as those with particular conditions ("My name is _____ and I am an alcoholic"), few people have practical identities that come with clear implications for difficult medical decisions. That someone is a feminist Christian African-American economist tells us very little about whether she favors natural childbirth or would choose a promising but experimental treatment over the current standard therapy for a given condition.

If all there is to autonomy is adopting practical identities, HCPs have a great deal of leeway with respect to how to enable patients to fulfill these identities. It would seem to open the door for HCPs to choose all sorts of things for patients in the name of enabling them to exercise their practical identities. Here is a familiar example. My physician knows that

I prefer to avoid heart disease, and so informs me that he will be taking a sample of my blood to measure my cholesterol levels. I do not recall ever going through an explicit consent process for such an action.

But if each patient's adoption of a set of practical identities *is* the exercise of that patient's autonomy, why would we have to obtain informed consent at all? It would seem that all we really require in order to respect patient autonomy is confirmation of each individual's practical identities (and perhaps their relative weights so that we are prepared for potential conflicts). But of course there are reasons that we cannot abandon informed consent for specific procedures. In addition to the fact that patients and HCPs may disagree on acceptable levels of risk and the importance of ensuring that HCPs appreciate patients' chosen identities, patients are allowed to change their profile of practical identities. By asking for confirmation of consent, HCPs are often asking for confirmation of the patient's previous choices.

The detail and frequency with which the HCP should seek explicit informed consent for particular procedures will thus depend on the particulars of the HCP's relationship with the patient. The HCP who becomes more confident in understanding and appreciating the patient's practical identities and previous decisions will be more justified in exercising parentalism. This is consistent with the widely accepted maxim that consent is informed if it is consistent with the patient's previous decisions, as applied in Cassell's two cases cited earlier in this chapter. Any HCPs treating patients they hardly know or whose decisions have not fallen into a recognizable pattern have to be more active in making sure that their actions are consistent with the patients' goals and practical identities, and hence must be more active in seeking explicit informed consent.

One further point regarding practical identities: when we adopt a practical identity we take on a package of obligations many of which we may not have expected. I choose to be a parent, and then my child is born with unexpected impairments; I choose to be Samantha's faculty advisor, and then Samantha decides to become Samuel or to join an outlawed cult. We may change our practical identities, but it will not relieve us of some of the obligations we have accrued if they involve other people.

For instance, saying, "I no longer identify as this baby's father," does not make it permissible for me to abandon the baby. However, this obligation then ceases to be one of autonomy even though it began in an autonomous choice to adopt a practical identity. The principal source of the obligation becomes one of responsibility or beneficence.

Beneficence and Autonomy

The most dramatic dilemmas in medical ethics involve conflicts between beneficence and autonomy. The physician believes that it is in the patient's interest that her family be notified of her condition, but the patient refuses to give permission. The physician believes that the patient is a danger to himself unless admitted to a hospital, but the patient insists on returning home. The physician believes that the patient will die unless surgery is performed immediately, but the patient refuses consent. In such cases the physician must choose between helping the patient and respecting the patient's right to autonomy. This has been described as "... the conflict at the roots of bioethics ..." (Engelhardt 1996, 103). Grisso and Appelbaum (1998, 147) suggested that we "... think of a balance scale with 'autonomy' at one end and 'protection' at the other."

An important consequence of the system I have been developing is that, with respect to health of individuals qua persons, beneficence and autonomy do not compete. Rather, they converge. This can be seen through the following premises, which summarize the reasoning of this chapter and the preceding one. Here, 'health' refers to health of individuals qua persons:

1. If health is determined (at least in part) by the preferences of individuals, (specific) duties of medical beneficence are also determined by the preferences of individuals.

2. Health is determined by the preferences of individuals.

Therefore:

3. Duties of medical beneficence are determined by the preferences of individuals.

Therefore:

4. When we fulfill a duty of medical beneficence we are acting in accordance with the preferences of individuals.

5. Acting in accordance with the preferences of individuals is part of respecting autonomy.

Therefore:

6. When we fulfill a duty of medical beneficence, we fulfill part of a duty to respect autonomy.

Premise 1 is, in simplified form, the thesis of chapter 3 and premise 2 is one thesis of chapter 2. Premise 3 follows from 1 and 2. Premise 4 is understood to be a reasonable inference from premise 3 alone. Premise 5 is offered as a simple gloss on autonomy, and proposition 6, one of the points I want to make in this chapter, follows from 4 and 5. Acting in accordance with preferences of individuals is only part of respecting autonomy because there is a difference between acting in merely accordance with duty and acting from (out of) duty (Kant 1959). Doing the right thing for the wrong reasons (or by accident) is insufficient.

Parentalism and Autonomy

No discussion of autonomy is complete without a look at *parentalism.* Traditionally called "paternalism" or, more radically, "maternalism," parentalism is the practice of acting on behalf of an individual when that individual has not given permission.[19] Some theorists distinguish between personal and state parentalism. Instances of state paternalism include laws, such as those requiring that drivers be insured, that restrict the freedom of individuals in a way that serves the best interests of those same individuals or of groups to which they belong. Most HCPs tend to think of individual parentalism as applying only to actions that are actually contrary to a choice expressed by the patient—for instance, sedating and confining a suicidal patient who has declared an intention to leave the hospital in order to kill himself elsewhere. The sense in which I use the term is broader, and includes cases of presumed consent, in which it seems clear what the patient would choose were he or she conscious (or able to communicate).

What is good for the individual's health qua person is what the individual chooses or would choose—what would be the result of the individual's autonomous choice were he or she in a position of knowledge, ability, and time to make such a choice. As I noted above, we can understand the autonomous choices of individuals in terms of practical identities. Of course, not all of a person's choices are autonomous. In particular, a patient's choice will not be autonomous when she is incapacitated or unable to determine what course of action will be consistent with her practical identities. The most common case is that in which the patient does not have the information or experience necessary to make a given decision, such as which antibiotic to take to treat an infection. A decision made on behalf of a patient in such a situation is an exercise of parentalism. As parentalism describes what we do on behalf of other *persons*, we need not distinguish between parentalism with respect to health qua person and health qua organism. That said, parentalist actions usually preserve or restore health qua organism in the interest of supporting health qua person.

As a form of beneficence, parentalism is sometimes understood as competing with autonomy, as coming into play when autonomy is not in the patient's best interest. However, our discussion suggests that parentalism is about extending patient autonomy, not limiting it. This is because an action of medical beneficence will be consistent with the individual's practical identities.

Thinking of parentalism as a way to realize patient autonomy does have its pitfalls, however. One is the way it allows us to justify acting against the stated wishes of a patient by simply denying that the patient is exercising or in a position to exercise autonomy. Indeed, it is common for HCPs to judge patients incompetent when they refuse consent for treatment in accord with the standard of care. The reasoning is that if the patient does not agree to what the HCP holds to be consistent with beneficence, the patient could not be acting autonomously. After all, autonomous persons choose what is good for them. In an oft-repeated example, a patient is judged incompetent (lacking in autonomy) because he refuses treatment for a life-threatening condition. Then, perhaps as soon as fifteen minutes later, he agrees to treatment and the physician accepts this consent as valid to proceed. The patient who was not competent to *refuse* treatment a quarter hour ago is suddenly competent to *consent to* treatment.[20]

Aside from obvious inconsistencies in applying the label "incompetent," this example raises two troubling issues. First, although it is best for patients to exercise autonomy simply and purely, HCPs too often do not have or do not take the time to enable patients to make autonomous decisions even when this would be possible with some effort. Consent to the standard of care can often, perhaps even usually, be obtained by listening to the patient's fears, correcting the patient's false beliefs, or providing the patient with adequate information. Time invested in these activities is time that could be used to treat other patients. This is, of course, just a problem of obtaining informed consent.

Second, it is commonly presumed that what is good for the health of the patient qua organism determines the duty of medical beneficence. As the physician is the one with the most obvious authority on the subject of the health of human organisms, paraprofessionals, family members, and others involved are likely to defer to the physician's recommendation. The patient's voice is left out of the discussion except as an echo of the "medical" recommendation, and is not recognized except when the content he or she voices is the same as that being voiced by the HCP.

Although maximizing health qua organism is often the best we can do, it is important to recognize what we ought to be striving for in such situations; that is, ceteris paribus, maximizing the exercise of autonomy and, through this, maximizing health of patients qua persons.

Conclusion

Chapter 2 presented the Richman–Budson theory as embedded instrumentalist and claimed that it was an intrinsic normativity theory. We have now explained the way in which preference satisfaction theories of health carry intrinsic normativity—Kantian ways. Invoking the Kantian notion of humans as ends in themselves, we at once explain the normativity in embedded instrumentalist theories and justify valuing the health of individuals qua persons over the health of individuals qua organisms. At the same time, we suggest that the value of health qua organisms is instrumental—the health of organisms is good merely as a means to realizing the autonomous choices of persons.[21]

Has our Kantian explication of autonomy enabled us to avoid the objections outlined above, which claim to show that autonomy is not an ideal we should be reaching for? We will address this question in the next chapter as it relates to identities and goals in the medical context.

The overriding argument of this chapter and the preceding one is summarized above. The conclusion is that duties of medical beneficence for health of patients qua persons are the same (in practice if not in justification) as duties to respect patient autonomy. These duties are also, then, equivalent to duties of parentalism. Insofar as they involve respecting the practical identities of persons, they are also duties of respect for persons.[22]

5

Conclusion to Part II

In chapter 4 I stated that we should understand patient autonomy in terms of practical identities. As this concept was developed by Korsgaard, the practical identities each individual adopts determine a set of values and rules for action. As autonomy is exercised by freely accepting and acting on such values and rules, the healthcare professional's (HCP's) duty to respect and further patient autonomy is best fulfilled by developing an understanding of the patient's practical identities. The greater the HCP's understanding and appreciation of the patient's practical identities, the more confident the HCP can be that informed consent has been obtained and that chosen treatments are consistent with and promote the values inherent in those practical identities.

Given a preference-satisfaction view of health, we see that enabling a patient to realize his or her practical identities is enabling the patient to be healthy qua person and hence is an act of medical beneficence. By suggesting that autonomy be understood at the level of practical identities, I am able to defend a view in which beneficence and autonomy do not compete.

Beneficence and autonomy often seem to compete, however. This occurs, for example, when a patient has not established a set of practical identities, when the patient has adopted inconsistent practical identities, or when the patient fails to realize how chosen practical identities relate to facts about the world. In such cases, the patient has failed to do a good job of realizing a capacity for autonomy and of setting a profile establishing what counts as his or her medical (and other) good. Of course, beneficence and autonomy may seem to compete when beneficence is viewed in terms of health qua organism, and the patient's goals and situation are such that improving health qua organism is incompatible with improving health qua person.

This chapter attempts to wrap up or at least follow some of the loose ends left by our discussions earlier in part II. These include the relationship between the kind of goal talk that I want to encourage and outcomes-based medicine, incommensurability of goals, and application of my theory to children. I end this chapter by placing my treatment of ethics in the context of some recent relevant philosophical work. In part III I discuss more explicitly how my theory applies in practical arenas, with a focus on advance directives and on how we might prepare physicians and other HCPs to implement my concept of health.

Goals and Evidence-Based Medicine

The medical literature tends to treat patient goals as important to patient satisfaction and compliance with treatment recommendations. Also discussed is the role of patient goals in choosing which medical problems *as identified by HCPs* are to be addressed first. Indeed, in their discussion of "collaborative management of chronic illness," Von Korff et al. (1997, 1097) wrote of "patient-defined problems" and "medical problems diagnosed by physicians." This language suggests that problems defined by patients are not medical. A typical study involving health goals measures whether patients with a curtain condition are able to function in ways specified by a measure such as the Functional Independence Measure or the Katz Activities of Daily Living Index (cf. McDowell and Newell 1996). Thus, in a show of self-awareness, Rockwood, Stolee, and Fox (1993, 1114) wrote:

Goal setting is accomplished by a consensus of the team members, based on the clinical judgement of the various health professionals. To date, the goal-setting, while not ignoring patient's wishes, does not formally incorporate their preferences.

The study involved elderly patients, many of whom had cognitive impairment. However, they also had practical identities, histories of decision making, relationships, and so on. Current dementia does not erase past decisions and values.

Attention to the efficacy (and hence efficiency) of medicine has shifted focus to so-called evidence-based medicine. According to the *New York Times*, evidence-based medicine was one of the most influential ideas of the year 2001 (Hitt 2001). The program of evidence-based medicine is to subject accepted treatment procedures to empirical testing. It turned up some surprising results. The lesson physician Kevin Patterson (2002, 76) drew ". . . is that the conclusions doctors reach from clinical experience and day-to-day observation of patients are often not reliable." In fact, HCPs have been surprised by results of studies of the effectiveness of hormone-replacement therapy in preventing postmenopausal heart disease, the effectiveness of mammograms in screening for breast cancer, and the like.

The hope is that evidence-based medicine will improve the effectiveness of health care while lowering costs by limiting the application of ineffective procedures. It holds out the promise of a standard of care based in good science rather than in local traditions or "standards of the community." Evidence-based medicine is also understood in a sense as defrocking the physician; when data are available to literate patients and announced on the nightly news, physicians no longer have exclusive access to the golden keys that unlock the mysteries of health problems.[1]

Moving data out of the HCP's head and into the public realm effects a democratization that enables patient autonomy:

The instant the practitioner stops saying, "I think you should take this therapy," and starts saying, "The evidence is that this therapy will work this percent of the time, with these complications, this frequently; what do *you* want to do?" then the power hierarchy of doctor over patient is collapsed, and autonomy is assigned to the patient. (Patterson 2002, 77)

Patterson's rosy portrayal of this more "scientific" approach to medicine is common, although perhaps more among nonphysicians than among physicians. One worries, however, about whether patients are sufficiently capable and confident in their processing of outcomes data that turning decisions over to them succeeds in supporting autonomy in any meaningful sense.

Sandra J. Tanenbaum framed the emergence of outcomes research and its application as evidence-based medicine differently. She contrasted the probabilistic reasoning of outcomes research with the deterministic knowledge sought by traditional bench science:

Outcomes research . . . creates information about what is likely to work, for whatever reason. By subjecting "real-life" data to rigorous analysis, outcomes research would seem to maximize a doctor's chances of doing the right thing. (Tanenbaum 1994, 61)

Whereas traditional medical science identifies causes and mechanisms that can be cited as explanations of disease and manipulated to effect changes, outcomes research identifies populations and probabilities. The difficulty is that HCPs tend to treat individuals, not populations. To argue from evidence that treatment T is effective 70 percent of the time for a given population to the conclusion that treatment T has a 70 percent chance of being effective for a specific member of that population is fallacious. It is to commit the fallacy of division. (The population of my household is 50 percent feline, but the likelihood that I will turn out to be feline is distinctly less than 50 percent.)

Tanenbaum found that even physicians who accepted the legitimacy of outcomes research were hesitant to apply it to the treatment of individual patients. She related a particularly telling conversation in which a physician considered whether he would follow outcomes-based treatment guidelines in a case in which they were contrary to his own judgment. The case involved the likelihood of success of kidney transplantation in an elderly man:

The physician insisted that his decision would stand—after all, perhaps the studies had overlooked an important subgroup of elderly renal patients, and besides, *he knew just how this patient's body worked and how kidney transplantation in this patient's body would succeed.* (Tanenbaum 1994, 66, emphasis hers)

We are not at this point very interested in the way physicians actually reason, but this anecdote is helpful. It is helpful because, I would hazard, most would consider the physician to be acting rightly and rationally in basing his treatment recommendation on knowledge of the patient even in the face of contrary outcomes for a relevant population.

In short, evidence-based medicine, in which treatment is determined on the basis of outcomes research, is problematic because it applies to individuals data aggregated from populations. It also draws conclusions about medical outcomes based on goals set by researchers rather than on goals set by patients. Given a theory of health such as mine, individuals must assess whether the outcome considered successful in a study would be an improvement given the individual's particular goals,[2] not just standard goals.

This is not to say that aggregated data yield no important and useful information. Despite the problematic application of outcomes research, if health measurements are made too individually they will not yield the generalizations that clinicians must rely on when making treatment decisions for each patient. These generalizations can be particularly crucial when the clinician has little or no direct experience of the condition, population, or individual. However, the data must be *applied* in a way that takes individuals and individuality into account.

Outcomes for Individuals

Although much of the literature on patient goals is rather flat-footed, applying standard measures uniformly across populations of patients with diverse interests, histories, and needs, some authors recognize that assessing the health status of an individual patient may be a more subtle, individual matter. Bioethicists and medical practitioners recognize the importance of identifying and supporting patient goals, and of facilitating clarification of these goals:

> . . . once it is recognized that significant medical decision making may confront a person with new information that challenges his or her self-understanding and capacity to exercise self-direction, processes that assist the person to reexamine, when possible, one's preferences, goals, values, and so on may better assist autonomous choice than clear information provision alone. (Dodds 2000, 231)

Dodds suggests a sense of autonomy richer than simply presenting likely outcomes and asking the patient to decide what to do. She recognizes, of course, that counseling is not always practical in medical situations, but notes it as an ideal.

Some of the literature on rehabilitation is also in tune with the ideas I am defending. Margaret G. Stineman understands the purpose of rehabilitation in terms of the life activities that are meaningful to the patient. She describes rehabilitation as ". . . a set of philosophies, treatments, and therapies that, when combined with natural recovery, are intended to enhance patients' potential for participating in meaningful life experiences" (Stineman 2001, 148).

She advocates assessing outcomes of rehabilitation therapy in terms of participation in meaningful life experiences rather than in terms of restored or improved physiological function. Maximizing physiological function does not necessarily yield the best outcome for a course of rehabilitation:

> Although the physiologic stage suggests common patterns of recovery, the trajectories of functional recovery that are most meaningful to participation in life experiences will differ among people and do not follow the same laws.[3] (Stineman 2001, 157–58)

This distinction between physiological functioning and ability to participate in the life experiences that are most meaningful to the individual closely parallels my distinction between health of the individual qua organism and health of the individual qua person. But when she remarks, "The objective is to use medical knowledge to empower the patient so that he or she can make the best choices" (Stineman 2001, 157), Stineman borders on suggesting that participation in valued life experiences is not a medical issue but an issue of some other sort (perhaps of ethics or of quality of life). I want to be clear that I consider my concept of the health of individuals qua persons to be just as much a medical concept as is my concept of health of individuals qua organisms.

Stineman is not the only researcher to find that individual members of the same patient population often have different health-related goals. Based on a concept of health-related quality of life (HRQOL), Gorbatenko-Roth et al. (2001) observed differences among patients in the relative importance they assigned to different areas of functioning. They were unable to offer specific recommendations for operationalizing the application of HRQOL to individuals, however, and noted that those with cancer in particular had difficulty expressing their preferences in response to direct questions about which domains of functioning they valued most (Gorbatenko-Roth et al. 2001). They conclude that "nonindividualized HRQOL measures" are acceptably accurate for *groups* of people when they include the three "primary domains" of physical functioning, emotional functioning, and role functioning. However, "At the individual level of analysis . . . a clinically feasible method of identifying a person's intrinsic domain preferences is needed before the conceptual findings can be utilized practically" (Gorbatenko-Roth et al. 2001, 140).

Because of diversity among patients, studies of patient goals that aggregate data from groups of participants provide only a rudimentary starting point for actual treatment.

A study asking what people with MS wanted and expected from health care services concluded:

People with MS display a wide variation in their preference for services and unmet needs. Information about management (both conventional and unconventional), relevant tailored advice and access to appropriately skilled professionals should be feasible components of high quality care. This work has highlighted the value of involving people with MS in the identification of their preferences. . . . (Somerset et al. 2001, 29)

These conclusions are in line with my suggestion that a patient's goals often have to be explored and clarified before decisions can be made concerning what will best serve the health of the patient qua person. Data showing the diversity of patient goals and values help us to see that medical beneficence is about more than improving physiological functioning. As I contend, improving physiological functioning is likely to improve health of the patient qua organism, but promoting health of the patient qua person requires choosing therapies in light of understanding the patient's practical identities.

Other studies showed that goals of individual patients commonly change over time. Note that it is possible for aggregated data to be stable on retesting even when data provided by most of the individual participants have changed. Kohut et al. (1997) offer precisely such an example with the goals of HIV-infected patients. Whereas previous studies concluded that individual treatment preferences suffer little change over time, the analysis was in fact generalized over groups and did not track individual respondents (Kohut et al. 1997, 124). The stability of aggregated data masked significant instability in the preferences of individual members of the group:

There were significantly more people with any change in preferences (80 percent versus 63 percent) and more changes in preferences (27 percent versus 15 percent) at the first re-interview (about six months after the initial interview) than could be accounted for by changes related to the poor test-retest reliability of the AD [advance directive]-HIV questionnaire (measured within five days of the initial interview). (Kohut et al. 1997, 131)

These are important findings. The suggestion that medicine should be practiced on individual patients (or families) one at a time seems a platitude, as does the suggestion that HCPs should not assume patients' goals to remain the same forever. However, in the face of the rising influence of evidence-based medicine and outcomes research, which encourage HCPs to treat individual patients based on data aggregated from large studies, we may yet have to keep this suggestion in the forefront of discussions of patient care.

Incommensurability and Conflicting Goals

The topics we have been discussing raise issues of incommensurability. In this context, 'incommensurability' can take two related meanings. In one sense it refers to the way two or more goods valued by an individual may fail to be comparable; in the other, Kuhnian, sense, it refers to the idea that values and other concepts in one conceptual scheme or world view may fail to be comprehensible from another conceptual scheme or world view.

We might deny that choosing to improve cognitive functioning rather than mobility is like choosing between two procedures promising different levels of the same function or different risks and benefits in the same domain. This would be to say that these options are incommensurable in the sense of being *incomparable*. The following is a "rough definition of incomparability":

two items are incomparable if no positive value relation holds between them. (Chang 1997, 4)

A value relation holds between two items if a value measure can be applied to each item so that they may be compared. Thus value relations "are strictly three-place; x is better than y with respect to V, where V ranges over values" (Chang 1997, 5). The claim that mental functioning and physical functioning are incommensurable in the sense of being incomparable is the claim that no "covering value" exists by which both can be measured for comparison.[4]

In this way, a claim of incomparability is a rejection of the idea driving utilitarianism:

. . . the incommensurabilist holds . . . that for an ordinary agent to have a sane, reasonable outlook is not (in real life, in the real world) the same thing at all as it is for his outlook to amount to a preference ordering by reference to which the agent's well-considered actions may be seen as maximizing anything. (Wiggins 1997, 60)

The incommensurabilist about the values of individuals holds that some decisions are just brute choices about what to value rather than guesses about what will end up bringing more of some good by which the options might ideally have been measured.

Some theorists deny that values can be or are incommensurable. Elijah Millgram (1997) argues that whenever a choice is made, there must be some preference, and if there is some preference, there must be a way of comparing. This suggests that incommensurability is not an issue in everyday situations; the very act of choosing proves commensurability. But even if a covering value allows us to compare two options, we may still ask whether that value is relevant to the choice we face. In determining whether a given value is one we want to invoke, we may have to appeal to a value that allows us to evaluate covering values. This leaves us with a regress that does not end, ends in a brute fact about value, or ends in a brute choice of value.[5]

The structure of this trilemma is familiar from discussions of epistemic justification (see Audi 1998). One way to embrace an infinite regress option is by adopting a coherence theory of values.[6] In such a theory, we judge a value according to the other values that we have embraced. A choice that fits in, or coheres with, a given set of values is justified simply by its relationship to the set. If two values cohere equally with the set of established values, they are equally well justified. An agent can choose to adopt a value that fails to cohere with his or her current values by making appropriate adjustments to the other values adopted.

Coherentism about values makes sense, but does not solve the problem at hand. One must still face the choice of which values to start with, as well as all of the choices among competing values that cohere equally well with the initial set once adopted. Thus it seems that choosing one course of action over another must end in either a brute choice or a brute fact about what value is to be optimized. I have been urging that where the decision concerns the health of an individual qua person, the value comes from human choice. Without such choice, there is no fact about what goals or values must be pursued or promoted in order to improve the health of the individual.

The Richman–Budson theory embraces the idea that satisfaction of human preferences and goals is the good with which health is concerned, but does not tell us what the goals of individuals should be. Without taking a stand on incommensurability in *ethics*, I want to say that individuals can make choices even when they have no answer as to what value serves (or best serves) for comparing options. The gravity of embracing and building one's practical identities may indeed involve the kind of brute choices that incomparability forces, but that is just what it is to be in the world. Difficulties arise for HCPs when they must guess what choices a patient would make in situations where the patient has not already chosen and is not able to do so.

Things would be different if individuals' choices played no role, if some invariable feature constituted health for everyone (the Aristotelian, bio-statistical, and health qua organism concepts of health offer this sort of picture). In such a case, expected outcomes, conditions, and states would be commensurable—they could be compared with respect to how much of this invariable feature they yielded. We would still face choices concerning how to balance health and other goods, but the question of which states are healthy would not be dependent on choices of this character.[7]

Incommensurability in the sense of lack of translatability of value concepts and other concepts between world views is an issue of interpersonal communication and understanding rather than of choices facing one individual. Concerns are raised about incommensurability at various junctions of biomedicine, such as within scientific practice, in communication between researcher and clinician, and between clinician and patient. Each person's world view will shape how he or she understands and describes the world, and failure of complete understanding is to be expected (Veatch and Stempsey 1995, 265).

An interesting example of incommensurability across world views appears in an article by Richard Gunderman (2000, 10):

... individuals living in poverty may be more firmly grounded in the present, giving less thought to the morrow than health professionals, who by dint of character and long experience take delayed gratification for granted. To talk about the increased risk of heart disease and stroke decades down the road from failing to take anti-hypertension medicine today may have little effect, because the patient's temporal horizon may not extend that far. Perhaps the patient's sense of vulnerability is already fully engaged by the prospect of avoiding violent death on the way home from the hospital. . . . Other circumstances may have inculcated the view that they simply don't have much control over their lives.

Gunderman pointed out that HCPs and certain patient populations may have different attitudes toward the future based on different life experiences. However, in describing the HCP's long-term strategy as the product of "character" and "long experience" he exhibited incommensurability as well as he explained it. It may show as much character to respond as patients do to experiences very different from those of HCPs. The patients may have just as much experience, but experience that gives rational warrant to a different outlook. Gunderman suggested that their choices, which seem wrong-headed to HCPs, can be explained in ways that allow HCPs to avoid blaming the patients. He missed the further point that the idea that individuals of high character pursue delayed gratification may simply have no place in a world view justified by the experiences of some patient populations.

Incommensurability in this second sense does not put the kibosh on patients making decisions for themselves, on the claim that medical beneficence is determined by the goals and practical identities chosen by individuals. However, it is very likely to hinder many attempts by HCPs to understand patient goals and by patients to communicate their goals.

Have We Avoided Objections to Autonomy?

In chapter 4 we identified six objections to the concept of autonomy as it is developed and applied in the medical context. We may now consider how our reconstruction of autonomy fares in the face of these objections. This reconstruction need not meet every objection fully, but it must at least not be made to seem ridiculous in their light. Remember, as well, that I am offering autonomy, even in its close connection with my theory of health, as only a prima facie good that will sometimes be overridden by other goods in particular circumstances. (I do not offer arguments as to when, how, or why such overriding may be a factor.)

Objections Based on Rejection of Associated Values

The first objection states that autonomy tends to come with conceiving of the ideal decision maker as an atomistic individual rather than as a person embedded in a complex system of relationships and roles. This prompted the remark, "Traditional conceptions [of autonomy] are . . . masculinist conceptions" (Mackenzie and Stoljar 2000, 8–9). This sort of individualism is not a given in the reconstruction of autonomy based on practical identities. Of course, individuals may choose to adopt practical identities premised on independence, such as hermit, or rogue demon hunter. However, our reconstruction also allows for identities that are essentially tied into the interests and practices of others. In identifying as a parent, an individual takes on the interests of another; in identifying as a soldier or a violist in a symphony orchestra, an individual takes on an interest in acting as part of a group. Thus our conception of autonomy at least mitigates the effect of drawing in these questionable values.

Objections Based on Irrationality of Persons

The second objection concerns the requirement of rationality. Since people tend to be irrational in predictable and unpredictable ways, few actual decisions will satisfy the traditional concept of autonomy. The demands of our reconstructed notion are not as inflexible and strict as those of the traditional notion. In the traditional notion, each decision to act is another atomistic opportunity to contradict the maxims guiding one's previous actions. Insofar as adopting practical identities is adopting bundles of goals at once, the individual has less opportunity to create contradictions. We can understand a person's choices as autonomous and coherent at the level of practical identities even when he or she is singularly inept at choosing individual acts by which to pursue the identities. (Ineptitude of this sort is sometimes acknowledged with the moniker "schlemazel.")

Objections Based on Rejection of the Individual

These objections are based on the claim that the idea of an autonomous individual person is incoherent, that our very personhood is relational. In a strong version of this view, the term 'autonomous individual' does not refer to a possible entity in the actual world. A weaker version might make no explicit ontological claim, but yet hold that conceiving of persons as autonomous decision-making atoms is likely to lead us to choose to act in ways that are ethically impermissible. The weaker version does not connect with my account of autonomy itself, but suggests that promoting autonomy may be ethically troubling. The weaker version is thus a species of the first objection.

As noted, in my view the practical identity of individuals will generally but not necessarily include relationships and responsibilities to others. Those embracing the strong version of this objection say something even stronger. They claim that it makes no sense to speak of a person and her other-relating identities as if they were separable even conceptually. Nothing I will offer refutes this stronger version. Although the objection deserves careful attention, here I merely note it and assert that it is useful to speak and think about individuals even if this means idealizing a messy world.

Objections Based on the Nature of the Role of Patient

Patients are, by etymology and otherwise, passive rather than active. Indeed, one characteristically becomes a patient when experiencing failure of autonomy, inability to do what one chooses to do (Fulford 1989). Furthermore, patients are rarely in a position to have or develop a full understanding of the diagnoses and treatments they discuss with HCPs. These are important reasons for doubting that patient autonomy can play a significant role in decisions about medical care.

My view allows, even coheres with, this family of objections. I maintain that autonomy is not a matter of making one choice at a time, but rather of adopting practical identities—packages of rules for choosing how to act. We adopt these identities by acting in ways that fall into general patterns, by joining clubs, by establishing relationships, and so on. Of course, we have some freedom to pick and choose, to construct our practical identities according to our interests. We need not choose just from the selection of identities exhibited by individuals and communities around us; for instance, we can build a new way to be a parent or a friend. Our practical identities can guide our choices and the choices that are made for us even when our capacity is diminished.

When patients face difficult medical choices, their practical identities may offer little by way of guidance. This may be because (1) the options under consideration are equally good with respect to patients' values, (2) patients have no way to determine which option will best support their values, or (3) the options simply do not connect with any of the values already adopted by the patients. If (1) is the case, patients should be indifferent to the options; any choice is consistent with respecting their autonomy. If (2) is the case, the issue is one of epistemology; patients and HCPs must take their best guess as to which option best supports the patients' practical identities. Item (3) describes situations in which patients' practical identities do not address the choices at hand. If this is the case for a great many everyday choices, we may complain that the individual is not realizing the potential for autonomy and that it would be better, perhaps even obligatory, for the person to adopt additional practical identities.

I suggest that (3) is common in medical settings. When a pharmacist asks whether I prefer my prescription in bubblegum flavor or lemon-lime flavor, I can answer by considering my preferences. When a physician asks a woman whether she prefers to carry her pregnancy to term, she can answer by considering her present practical identities and whether to adopt one involving motherhood. Other choices might not connect with our established values. Do I want to have a small mole removed prophylactically, or observe it to see whether it might have to be removed later? This choice may require that I begin to establish a new practical identity—will I be the sort of patient who takes an aggressive, "pro-active" approach, or will I be a more conservative, wait-and-see type? Some patients have established their identities on this dimension, others have not.

Objections Based on the Claim That Many Patients Do Not Want Autonomy

Patients sometimes request that HCPs make choices for them. This is commonly described as giving up or refusing to exercise autonomy. This objection is subject to a technical rebuttal and a related substantive one. First, I expect that this phenomenon arises when patients cannot see how the choice they have to make relates to their practical identities. A choice that stands on its own, one that is part of no pattern of choices by the individual, will not be an exercise of autonomy strictly so called. That is the technical rebuttal: the choices that patients refuse to make would (in general, I suspect) not technically speaking be truly autonomous choices anyway.

Substantively, respect for patient autonomy may be an important factor in decisions for which the connection to the patient's established practical identities is obscure. Patients often just want to return to a state in which they fulfill the roles they have chosen and can resume making the kinds of decisions that they are comfortable with and that have meaning to them. Patients exercise their autonomy most fully when they are living the lives they have chosen. HCPs can show respect for patient autonomy by assisting in restoring or maintaining patients' abilities to live these lives, and this often means making decisions for patients.

Objections Based on Improper Application
As I stated in the last chapter, traditional notions of patient autonomy are invoked to cover many sins. Patients who request nonstandard treatment, or who simply disagree with a treatment recommendation, are declared incompetent to make autonomous choices on the basis of their apparent "irrationality." Those who refuse treatment through fear, mistrust, or misunderstanding may be left in serious condition out of respect for their "autonomy." These very real examples cause some to doubt the usefulness of autonomy as a practical ideal.

Indeed, the version of autonomy that I advocate introduces another type of misuse. In my reconstructed Kantian concept, a patient may end up looking at choices that are consistent with his or her practical identities but that seem foreign. Autonomy as I described it could lead to HCPs becoming overconfident in their ability to choose treatments for the patient even in the face of patient protest. The HCPs might defend their choices as consistent with the patient's practical identities even though the patient may not see that that is the case. The significance of this set of objections is that application of autonomy along the lines I have sketched should come in the context of carefully formulated safeguards.

Patient Incompetence

Competent patients can make medical requests that are ethically impermissible. Such requests have authority, but the HCP's duty of medical
beneficence that follows from this authority can be overruled by other
obligations. Patients can be competent but unable to communicate. They
may, for instance, be paralyzed due to injury or a disease such as ALS
(Lou Gehrig's disease). I maintain that in this case decisions should be
based on evidence of the patient's practical identities and previous decisions or, in the absence of such, that HCPs should act to maximize health
of the patient qua organism.

The discussion so far leaves unanswered concerns about certain forms
of patient incompetence. To be incompetent is to be unable to make decisions in a way that bears authority, that has legitimacy as part of medical
or other decisions. Patients can be incompetent in several ways.[8] They
may be simply unable to form preferences; comatose patients fall into
this category. For them, as for competent patients unable to communicate, HCPs should first look for evidence of past preferences and attempt
to maximize health qua organism in the absence of a clear answer
regarding health qua person.

Patients may be also be incompetent by virtue of being unable to
appreciate the simple or complex facts relevant to the decision at hand.
This can be due to insufficient education, low native intelligence, or
dementia. Many decisions are simply too complicated for intelligent,
educated patients to make for themselves without prohibitively time-con-
suming additional education. In such cases, the HCP must make a decision for the patient—that is, exercise parentalism. The HCP's level of
confidence that the decision accords with beneficent parentalism should
be proportioned to the likelihood, given available evidence, that the decision promotes the patient's goals and practical identities. This confidence
increases with greater understanding of the patient's goals and identities;
it decreases with greater risk that a treatment will have an undesirable
side effect or outcome.

An HCP who can confidently make a difficult decision for a patient
when that patient is unable to understand the intricacies of this decision
may proceed with patient assent. (I use the term "assent" rather than

"consent" because a patient cannot offer valid informed consent to a decision with respect to which he or she is incompetent.) An HCP facing a decision with low confidence can learn more about the patient to increase the confidence. The HCP can also do more to spread the burden of decision making by involving other surrogate decision makers and by increasing the patient's competence through education. In short, decreased confidence that a decision satisfies medical beneficence for a patient qua person calls for increased care before implementing that decision. James F. Drane (1984) defended a similar "sliding scale" approach to consent.

Those who are suicidal or who suffer from paranoia or narcissism may also be unable to appreciate relevant facts. Some suicidal patients, for instance, are unable to weigh facts about their present pain against facts about how they are likely to feel in the future. Other kinds of pain also tend to distort one's sense of the facts in a way that "discounts" the future.

Another example of inability to appreciate facts is seen in patients who understand relevant details in some sense but are unable to reason well about them. For them, the HCP may see a duty of medical beneficence that is incompatible with patients' stated requests. In a sense, the patient and HCP disagree about what the patient wants. The patient says "I want X," and the HCP says "No, you do not want X." Here, the HCP would ideally seek to determine what we, following Railton, call the patient's objectified subjective interest. (See chapter 2.) As with other types of incompetent patients, HCPs have an obligation to act in a way consistent with a carefully assessed level of confidence regarding patients' health interests.

We must, of course, be careful to avoid judging competent individuals to be incompetent. In our model, this will be particularly likely when someone changes practical identities. If rationality and (hence) autonomy require consistency, we will be suspicious when someone who has been a cautious driver for many years suddenly sells a Volvo station wagon to buy a motorcycle. We will want to call that person incompetent on the basis of irrationality, nonautonomous on the basis of inconsistent choices.[9] On the one hand, it seems an archetypal example of autonomy for someone to choose to hit the open road with exhaust pipes roaring. On the other hand, we want an explanation for the change. Did the person undergo some experience that can account for the change, such as a religious conversion or a financial inheritance?

Individuals sometimes change their values. At one time I did not like cabbage, but I do now. This does not make me incompetent. However, as we discussed in chapter 2, some sets of goals are inconsistent in ways that, should they be adopted, indicate incompetence. And, as discussed here, one may be incompetent by virtue of being unable to select means likely to promote one's chosen ends.

One could also adopt new practical identities in ways that do not bear authority. Changes based on delusions, intoxication, or misinformation, for instance, will not make legitimate claims on HCPs. The difficulty lies in assessing which choices are legitimate. This difficulty is especially challenging given a picture of autonomy according to which an individual's ability to choose freely is most solidly in evidence when values do not change at all, and in which any consistent set of practical identities is open for adoption. Various modes of inquiry may be applied to understand the patient's choice and to make sure that it reflects real values and coheres with the patient's beliefs and relevant facts about the world. In many cases, one will simply have to accept that the patient has changed his or her practical identities.

Although such changes do not make one irrational, practical identities become meaningless if they are changed too often. A patient whose practical identities are in constant flux must be said to have limited autonomy and only a vaguely determined health status qua person. What counts as constant flux is a matter of degree.

Conclusion: Respect for Persons

I have framed my treatment of medical ethics in terms of principles, noting that principles are to be checked against cases according to a sort of reflective equilibrium that was referred to as coherentism (Beauchamp and Childress 2001, 397ff). Although principles are often associated with a deontological approach to ethics,[10] I treated respect for patient autonomy and duties of medical beneficence in terms of satisfying patient goals and promoting patients' practical identities. In this way, my position on medical duties has important consequentialist strands.[11] However, I rejected views, such as utilitarianism, according to which there is only one relevant consequence. Instead, I identified duties of the HCP to promote patient health, where health of the patient qua person is understood in terms of outcomes that may be valued specifically by that patient. This is the embedded instrumentalist, or preference-satisfaction, approach that I have been defending. I maintain that HCPs' duties of medical beneficence are subject to conflict with other ethical duties.

The constellation of duties I described in part II can be understood as falling under a general concept of *respect for persons*. My presentation of autonomy in terms of practical identities rather than individual choices especially lends itself to being characterized in this way. The duty to respect autonomy as reconstructed here is a duty to promote the identities of the individual rather than to follow each choice considered by itself. Others, including Beauchamp and Childress, understood duties to honor patient autonomy in terms of respect for persons.[12] No harm is done in thinking of it this way. However, I prefer to emphasize autonomy because, in my understanding, an important strand in thinking about the value of persons is conceptually based in the ability of persons (considered as an idealized class) to exercise autonomy. Thus autonomy is prior to respect for persons.

Postscript to Part II: Paul Bloomfield's Moral Realism

In his book *Moral Realism*, Paul Bloomfield (2001) argues for a realism about moral goodness by defending a realism about health and claiming that goodness allows of parallel treatment. We must be realists about health, he claims, because there is a definite difference between the extremes of health—being alive and being dead:

... no properties are more deserving of realism than those of being alive and being dead, and since the difference between them is one of healthiness, we cannot be other than realists about health without also denying that life differs from death. (Bloomfield 2001, 32)

Health is understood here as fitness or ability to survive. This conception has room for disagreement as to which among equally fit states count as healthy.[13] "And here we find health's compossibility with relativism" (Bloomfield 2001, 35). Disagreements over which states are healthy could arise from disagreement over facts concerning the relative fitness of states or concerning preferences among equally fit states. If the disagreement centers around something else, it is not a disagreement about (physical) health. The existence of states that are functionally equivalent with respect to fitness allows Bloomfield to embrace both realism and relativism with respect to health and health assessments.

Bloomfield uses these findings about the character of health to show how moral realism is consistent with relativism about goodness. He continues the analogy to propose that moral epistemology is isomorphic with the epistemology of health. Along the way, he claims that:

Both [goodness and healthiness] entail purposes that are given to us in virtue of being the kinds of creatures we are and establish standards by which we may evaluate what we ought to do. (Bloomfield 2001, 42)

He is not claiming that ethics and health are the same. He contends that health is a good different from moral goodness, as do I. But we can now see how his view differs from mine.

Bloomfield holds that the moral status of an action is not determined by the contingent values of society or individuals. Instead,

. . . it is our nature as *Homo sapiens* that fixes the constraints on what counts as good, not our moral practices, which can be only more or less efficacious at helping us to live well. (53)

This is a form of Aristotelianism, as I have characterized it. As Aristotle himself observed, it is consistent with the view that ". . . healthiness is a property that is relativized to both species and individuals" (Bloomfield 2001, 39). Bloomfield's account resonates with the Richman–Budson theory of health qua organism, but not with the concept of health qua person.

III

Clinical Connections

6

Advance Directives[1]

Developments in medical technology make it possible to keep individuals alive even when they are gravely ill, have extremely diminished capacities, and would die without this technology. Because such interventions can be the only factors sustaining the life of individuals when their capacities are reduced to nearly null, their use does not always seem mandatory. Situations occur in which sincere disagreement may arise as to whether keeping someone alive confers a benefit.

Consider the English patient of March 2002. Miss B was paralyzed from the neck down after a blood vessel in her neck ruptured. She depended on a ventilator because she could not breathe for herself. Her doctors judged that her chance of recovering from this paralysis was approximately 1 percent. Miss B sued to be allowed to die. Dame Elizabeth Butler Sloss, the High Court judge who heard the case, ruled in favor of Miss B, judging that Miss B had the "necessary mental capacity" to refuse life-sustaining treatment (BBC News 2002). Dame Elizabeth said, "One must allow for those as severely disabled as Miss B, for some of whom life in that condition may be worse than death."

This case is a very robust example of an apparently competent patient asserting her autonomy in the context of a broad understanding of what makes her life worth living. When a medical intervention such as a ventilator or feeding tube is required to keep an individual alive but the life is of marginal quality, we ideally consult the patient to determine whether the artificial method is "worth it."

The difficulty, of course, is that such cases are characteristically ones in which the patient is unable to express preferences or is not competent to give informed consent. This sets up a situation in which parentalism seems appropriate—the patient cannot decide, so the field is open for the health care professional (HCP) to step in and decide on the patient's behalf. However, as the discussion in part II shows, to act consistently with medical beneficence toward the patient qua person, the HCP must understand the patient's values. That is, the HCP ought to choose a course of treatment that will maximize the patient's ability to fulfill his or her goals and practical identities. As goals and practical identities vary widely, the HCP must understand the patient as an individual in order to choose a treatment that maximizes health of the patient qua person. Lacking access to this understanding, it is permissible for the HCP to aim to maximize health of the patient qua organism. However, this latter medical beneficence can run counter to what would ideally embody respect for persons and respect for autonomy. Health care advance directives have the potential to address these issues.

The term *health care advance directive* applies to traditional living wills (that specify preference for life support treatments and end-of-life care), health care power of attorney documents, and other statements of preferences intended to serve as guides to health care at some future time when the individual is unable or incompetent to decide or to communicate a decision. The American Medical Association (2002) describes advance directives as follows:

A health care advance directive is a document in which you give instructions about your health care if, in the future, you cannot speak for yourself. You can give someone you name (your "agent" or "proxy") the power to make health care decisions for you. You also can give instructions about the kind of health care you do or do not want.

Through a health care advance directive, individuals can increase the likelihood that their preferences will be respected. The primary impetus for advocating advance directives is respect for patient autonomy coupled with respect for persons.[2] These documents can increase the likelihood that the care given to patients when they become incompetent will satisfy the HCP's duty of medical beneficence with respect to health of patients qua persons.

In the following sections I examine some ideas from the literature and sample advance directives. We will see that documents widely used in the United States are not constructed to maximize patient autonomy where autonomy is understood as I advocated in part II. I offer some preliminary suggestions for a more successful way of constructing advance directives, and propose that, properly constructed, they have the potential to maximize autonomy, beneficence, and *health*. My reasoning is an application of the discussion in chapter 4.

A Standard Medical Advance Directive Document

In 1990, the United States Congress enacted the Patient Self-Determination Act (PSDA), part of that year's Omnibus Budget Reconciliation Act. The goal of the PSDA is to increase the numbers of patients who understand their rights and exercise them by completing appropriate advance directives. The primary methods of implementation are requiring health care facilities to develop literature about patient rights and advance directives, and requiring these facilities to ask each patient on admission whether he or she has an advance directive.

A look at the brochures on advance directives provided to patients at several Pennsylvania hospitals reveals closely similar content, taken from Pennsylvania Consolidated Statutes (2002)[3]:

Sample Declaration

I, _____, being of sound mind, willfully and voluntarily make this declaration to be followed if I become incompetent. This declaration reflects my firm and settled commitment to refuse life-sustaining treatment under the circumstances indicated below.

I direct my attending physician to withhold or withdraw life-sustaining treatment that serves only to prolong the process of my dying, if I should be in a terminal condition or in a state of permanent unconsciousness.

I direct the treatment be limited to measures to keep me comfortable and to relieve pain, including any pain that might occur by withholding or withdrawing life-sustaining treatment.

In addition, if I am in the condition described above, I feel especially strong about the following forms of treatment:

I ( ) do ( ) do not want cardiac resuscitation.

I ( ) do ( ) do not want mechanical respiration.

I ( ) do ( ) do not want tube feeding or any other artificial or invasive form of nutrition (food) or hydration (water).

I ( ) do ( ) do not want blood or blood products.

I ( ) do ( ) do not want any form of surgery or invasive diagnostic tests.

I ( ) do ( ) do not want any kidney dialysis.
I ( ) do ( ) do not want antibiotics.

I realize that if I do not specifically indicate my preference regarding any of the forms of treatment listed above, I may receive that form of treatment.

OTHER INSTRUCTIONS

I ( ) do ( ) do not want to designate another person as my surrogate to make medical treatment decisions for me if I should be incompetent and in a terminal condition or in a state of permanent unconsciousness.

Name and address of surrogate (if applicable):

_____.

Name and address of substitute (if surrogate designated above is unable to serve):

_____.

I ( ) do ( ) do not want to make an anatomical gift of all or part of my body, subject to the following limitations, if any:

_____.[4]

The statute indicates that advance directives need not conform to the sample, but since it is offered in the statute and reproduced by hospitals, I will treat it as standard (at least for Pennsylvania).

The text in the statute is reasonable in many ways. It is specific, it includes options that can be clearly understood by HCPs, and it will generally be easy to determine whether an advance directive in this form is being followed by HCPs. However, several features make it less than ideal. For instance, it discusses one type of situation in which the patient is incompetent and dying or permanently unconscious. This is not the only circumstance in which an advance directive could be useful. Although Miss B was neither dying nor permanently unconscious, an advance directive completed before she became paralyzed may have facilitated her case by giving further support to her claim that her choice to die was autonomous.

In our understanding of autonomy, individuals exercise autonomy by establishing and continuing patterns of action that express their values and practical identities. They do this by making decisions that are consistent across similar or otherwise related instances. For most of us, the thinly sketched example we are asked to consider in the standard advance directive document is sufficiently different from those we face in living our lives that we have no clear way to determine just what decision would count as consistent with the arc of decisions and actions established by our other choices.[5] (We can think of an individual's choices and actions as forming an arc in the sense that, as with a ball that has been hit or thrown, the earlier moments of the arc allow us to anticipate the later moments.) Of course, many individuals have chosen to write, protest, or act in other ways that determine a position, even a practical identity that is relevant to the example. However, if this decision fails to connect with our other decisions, the choices generated will fail, strictly speaking, to qualify as autonomous.

Furthermore, patients may fail to understand the medical procedures listed. Most (but not all) advance directive brochures containing the above text offer brief definitions of terms. But it is easily imaginable that a patient may fail to appreciate what is involved in a procedure such as kidney dialysis even given an accurate but simple explanation, typically along the lines of "kidney dialysis is a mechanical procedure that removes waste from the blood."

The sample declaration is primarily an opt-out document. That is, it offers patients the opportunity to refuse treatment that they can otherwise expect. This allows HCPs to pursue health of the individual qua organism where they have no way to determine what would count as health for the individual qua person.

However, it is unclear just when the provisions of the advance directive kick in. The document specifies that it applies to "the circumstance indicated," namely, one in which the patient is incompetent and ". . . in a terminal condition or in a state of permanent unconsciousness." A significant issue concerns what counts as a terminal condition. The wording suggests that one is in a terminal condition if treatment "serve[s] only to prolong the process of . . . dying." Although I am neither very old nor very pessimistic, I do not find it easy to distinguish between processes of living (after, say, puberty) and processes of dying. My morning vitamins extend my life. Is this because they prolong my dying or because they push the start of the dying process farther into the future? Because I do not at the moment see a principled way to distinguish between the two, I do not see a principled way to determine when the provisions of Pennsylvania's standard health care advance directive are to be implemented.

I do allow, however, that clear, paradigmatic cases will exist. Perhaps other cases can be assessed by their relation to the paradigmatic ones.

Rebecca Dresser, Ezekiel and Linda Emanuel, and others raised more general concerns about the efficacy and appropriateness of medical advance directives as a means of preserving and respecting patient autonomy. Dresser questioned whether the documents are being respected,[6] and even whether patients who have such documents want and expect them to be followed. She noted data suggesting that many individuals who make advance directives do so on the assumption that their proxies and physicians will not follow their instructions if these others believe the instructions to be unwise in the situation (Dresser 1994, S4). Thus she wondered what the directives are intended to accomplish:

Is the goal to help people "feel better" about their futures as incompetent, seriously ill patients? Is it to encourage them to acknowledge and take responsibility for events that are often painful to anticipate? Is the goal to allow them to give coherence to their lives by charting a death that fits their current self-image? (Dresser 1994, S4)

Several important reservations arose concerning whether the PSDA will result in the most ethically sound decisions and documents:

Among these reservations are that (1) admission to a health care facility is not an optimal time to introduce advance care planning; (2) the PSDA does not involve the patient's physician in advance care planning; and (3) there is no funding for mandated public education on advance care planning. (Emanuel et al. 1993, 619)

These concerns address the implementation of the act rather than the text of any document. However, they draw our attention to a variety of issues relevant to both implementation and content of the advance directive. Elsewhere, these authors addressed the text directly.[7]

The Emanuels' Medical Directive

People may find it difficult to anticipate situations in which an advance directive would be used for them (Emanuel and Emanuel 1989, 3291). This concern is along the same lines as the one that the examples described for standard advance directives (e.g., in Pennsylvania statute) do not connect with the arc of the individual's other choices in a way that makes choices the individual could make about these examples strictly speaking autonomous. To address this concern, patients might be presented with detailed descriptions of possible "illness scenarios and treatment options" to help them develop precise preferences that can be expressed in an advance directive (Emanuel and Emanuel 1989, 3291).

The Emanuels (1989) offered a model of advance directive that puts this suggestion to work. Four scenarios, twelve treatment options, and four attitude options are presented in a grid. For each scenario, the individual is asked to consider a list of treatments consisting of cardiopulmonary resuscitation, mechanical breathing, artificial nutrition and hydration, major surgery, kidney dialysis, chemotherapy, minor surgery, invasive diagnostic tests, blood or blood products, antibiotics, simple diagnostic tests, and pain medications, "even if they dull consciousness and indirectly shorten life." For each option in each scenario the individual can choose among four attitudes: I want this treatment if I am in a situation like the one described, I do not want this treatment if I am in a situation like the one described, I am undecided as to whether I want this treatment if I am in a situation like the one described, or I want this treatment tried and continued only if it results in clear improvement in my health status.[8]

This medical directive is open to most of the objections I raised against the Pennsylvania statute. Even when we describe possible scenarios fully and offer enough carefully chosen ones to cover likely possibilities, the situations considered are still ones that few people completing advance directives have faced before. In the terms of a traditional Kantian conception of autonomy, we must say that if we have not made choices about a type of situation (developed maxims and rules regarding them), the choices we make will not be autonomous (strictly speaking) because they will not be instances of *laws*. In the terms of the modified Korsgaardian Kantian concept of autonomy, the decisions asked for are simply not the kind that most people make as they go about their ordinary lives. The standard forms do not reflect the true medium of autonomy, the ways in which we embrace rules and obligations—practical identities.

The Values History and an AMA Booklet on Advance Directives

A booklet sponsored by the American Medical Association (AMA 2002) entitled "Shape Your Health Care Future with Health Care Advance

Directives" suggests that patients may want to create what they call a Values History. This reflects thinking among bioethicists that can be traced back to the 1970s[9]:

> In doing a Values History, you examine your values and attitudes, discuss them with loved ones or advisors and write down your responses to questions such as:
>
> • How do you feel about your current health?
> • How important is independence and self-sufficiency in your life?
> • How do you imagine handling illness, disability, dying, and death?
> • How might your personal relationships affect medical decision-making, especially near the end of life?
> • What role should doctors and other health professionals play in such decisions?
> • What kind of living environment is important to you if you become seriously ill or disabled?
> • How much should the cost to your family be a part of the decision-making process?
> • What role do religious beliefs play in decisions about your health care?
> • What are your thoughts about life in general in its final stages: your hopes and fears, enjoyments and sorrows?

The idea of values being embedded in or arising out of an individual's history is very much in the spirit of my theory of autonomy. An individual's values and identities are bundles of the rules by which she governs her life. These rules, though flexible, changing, and sometimes indeterminate, are guideposts for determining what choices count as autonomous. As I argued in part I, they are also the guideposts for determining what treatment decisions contribute to the health of the individual qua person.

As others described it, ". . . the Values History enhances the autonomy of the patient in a way that present advance directives do not. . . ." It does this ". . . by clarifying for the health care team the patient's expressed values underlying decisions to be carried out when decision making by the patient is no longer possible" (Doukas and McCullough 1991, 145). Values clarification by the patient can aid HCPs and health care institutions as they face the uncertainties that tend to accompany advance directives (Doukas and McCullough 1991, 145).

Doukas and McCullough proposed a Values History with two parts: "(1) an explicit identification of values, and (2) the articulation of advance directives based on the patient's values" (1991, 146). The Values History promotes autonomy generally by helping patients to think about how medical decisions that they do or may face connect with their practical identities. It holds the promise of extending patient autonomy and maximizing health of the patient qua person by making it more likely that medical interventions will be consistent with the patient's practical identities and hence will enable the patient to reach or strive for his or her goals.

The sample advance directive offered by Doukas and McCullough offers a list of common values, and instructs the patient to circle those "that are important to your definition of quality of life." The options listed include, "I want to maintain my capacity to think clearly," and "I want to be treated in accord with my religious beliefs and traditions." Space is provided for "other values or clarification of values above." It also asks for the patient's preference with respect to "length of life versus quality of life" (Doukas and McCullough 1991, 151). The second part of the document addresses specific treatments. For each decision regarding cardiopulmonary resuscitation (CPR), being put on a ventilator, and the rest, the document asks not only whether the patient wants to receive such treatment (yes, no, or on a trial basis "to determine effectiveness using reasonable medical judgment") (151), but also *why*.[10]

The AMA booklet[11] actually offers three ways of approaching advance directives. One is by doing a Values History. This can be an exercise for clarifying action preferences for one or more instances, or can be put in written form to serve as the advance directive document itself. Another is by identifying goals: ". . . you can make your preferences clear by stating your goals for medical treatment. What do you want treatment to accomplish?" Such goals can help caregivers determine when a given treatment is futile with respect to the patient's wishes, but this can be operational only when patients are aware that they are candidates for treatment.

Finally, the booklet offers a standard form on which an individual can indicate preferences based on outcomes. Thus the wording includes ". . . I do not want to receive treatment, including nutrition and hydration, when the treatment will not give me a meaningful quality of life" (AMA 2002). The declaration is completed by putting a check mark beside descriptions of outcomes that are not consistent with a "meaningful quality of life" for that individual.

The AMA's sample advance directive is thus different from the wording in the other documents we have examined. Wording in the Pennsylvania statute asks us to take the outcome as given (impending death or a permanent unconscious state) and indicate which treatments are unacceptable; the wording of the advance directive form in the AMA booklet takes the treatment as given and asks us to indicate which outcomes are unacceptable. The Emanuels's medical directive is much more comprehensive than either one. Not only does it allow us to opt out, it allows us to accept, reject, or accept provisionally many possible treatments with respect to four different expected outcomes. However, only the Values History allows patients to express their preferences in terms grounded in choices that they have already made as they have built their lives.

Balancing Clarity and Validity

I hope it is obvious that, in my view, the Values History and goals specification described in the AMA booklet and by Doukas and McCullough constitute the ideal way for patients to communicate information relevant to the provision of appropriate care. The two combined engage the individual in thinking not only about past choices (the history of one's values) but also about goals for the future—the full arc of one's choices. However, such documents may be too long and difficult or time consuming to digest when decisions must be made. Thus it seems appropriate to have a document that communicates both the kind of information that is easily digestible by HCPs (along the lines of the Emmanuels's medical directive and the second part of Doukas and McCullough's) and more subtle information about patient values and goals.

The Doukas and McCullough directive goes a long way toward collecting this information. I suggest three additional questions for collecting important information that is unlikely to be revealed by any of the documents mentioned so far:

1. Each person plays many roles in life. What aspects of your identity are important to you? Which of your roles do you see as essential to making your life worth living?

2. What abilities and activities are most important to you? Which of the things that you do are such that your life might not be worth continuing if you could not do them?

3. In many situations, outcomes of medical procedures can be uncertain. Some medical procedures that offer great potential benefit also carry great risk. How comfortable are you with risk? In general, are you willing to risk bad outcomes when there is hope of great benefit?

Obviously, the first asks the patient to identify central practical identities and the second asks after goals. Attitudes concerning risk identified by responses to number 3 are very important and not usually included in advance directives. Risk and probability are extremely difficult for most people to appreciate, but some are more risk averse than others. This information can be essential to determining appropriate care.

Implementation

Ambiguous directives can be expected, but even where one states clear preferences for unambiguous situations, implementation can still be fraught with difficulties. The following discussion addresses several problems that arise in implementing these documents.

When Physicians Refuse to Honor Requests

Patients have a right to request and refuse treatments according to their values. To HCPs, these requests may seem outrageous or immoral. What then?

HCPs have duties that others do not have. These duties arise out of their status as members of a profession and out of their relationships to their individual patients. I do not think that this relationship need be made formal in a contract (any more than the parent-child relationship need be) to generate obligations.

It is characteristic of the HCP's role to act on behalf of others. This is an important factor in determining the duties of HCPs. For instance, Howard Brody (1989) suggested an ideal of "transparency" in decision making by physicians. That is, when HCPs make a decision on behalf of or with regard to treatment of patients, they should make their reasoning perfectly clear to the appropriate party (ideally a competent adult patient). This strikes me as a strict duty in situations in which the prognosis will not suffer from delay for discussion and in which there is a competent responsible party. It is a duty that serves patient autonomy insofar as it provides for informed consent or informed refusal of treatment.

Pellegrino concluded that physicians have a duty to take on the interests and goals of patients as their own, much as one does for a friend. This is very much like what I have been defending in terms of respecting patients' practical identities. Our ordinary duty is only to respect practical identities; the HCP's duty to patients is to embrace and further the patient's practical identities in the medical context (using medically relevant expertise, etc.). This duty, however, is a prima facie duty. For instance, it is limited to permissible identities. That is, the HCP does not have a duty to embrace and further a patient's practical identity when that practical identity is that of a rapist or is otherwise reprehensible. This duty might also be limited by issues of distributive justice. If other patients are receiving only minimal care, promoting the banker's identity as a competitive golfer may have to wait.

In addition, it often happens that patients make requests or refusals inconsistent with their practical identities. This happens as a result of insufficient knowledge, fear, and so on. The HCPs do not have a duty to follow such requests or refusals, choices that are "inauthentic" (see Ganzini and Lee 1993). I do not pretend that it is easy to tell the difference between an inappropriate decision and a revision of one's practical identities. In addition, situations may exist in which there is no fact of the matter about which practical identities the patient has embraced. In these instances transparent reasoning on the part of the HCP can be particularly helpful because it gives the patient an opportunity to communicate whether the reasoning seems friendly or alien. (More on the transparency standard in the next chapter.)

Perhaps most contentious is the situation in which an HCP refuses to further one of the patient's core goals or identities on the basis of a value conflict. Disagreements about how best to promote or pursue the patient's goals can be worked out, but an HCP might refuse to give treatment on the basis that it is inconsistent with the *HCP's* practical identities. Refusing to take on the patient's goal as one to pursue is different from taking on the patient's goal and not acting on it due to overriding factors. Where an HCP refuses to consider a patient's stable, central, considered goal as among factors to be taken seriously, we must consider whether the HCP is guilty of abandoning the duty of medical beneficence. After all, promoting the patient's goals is improving the patient's health qua person. Also at issue with such refusals are the HCP's duties to respect persons, to be trustworthy, and to respect patient autonomy.

An HCP who refused to take an established patient's goal as prima facie motivating for unspecifiable or merely aesthetic reasons would indeed be neglecting a duty of medical beneficence. An HCP who refused to take an established patient's goal as prima facie motivating due to ethical objections is in essence weighing the duty of medical beneficence against other duties and deciding that it is impermissible to follow the duty of medical beneficence with such a patient at such a time. Considered choices of this sort should be accepted.

Several states have statutes recognizing the possibility that HCPs might object to the content of an advance directive. Consider, for instance, the following from the Pennsylvania statute:

> If an attending physician or other health care provider cannot in good conscience comply with a declaration [advance directive] or if the policies of the health care provider preclude compliance with a declaration, the attending physician or health care provider shall so inform the declarant, or, if the declarant is incompetent, shall so inform the declarant's surrogate, or, if a surrogate is not named in the declaration, shall so inform the family, guardian or other representative of the declarant. The attending physician or health care provider shall make every reasonable effort to assist in the transfer of the declarant to another physician or health care provider who will comply with the declaration. (Pennsylvania Consolidated Statutes 2002).[12]

Requiring that the HCP take reasonable steps to find an appropriate replacement professional is one way to recognize the importance of the duty of medical beneficence for patients qua persons.

When Patients Demand Futile Care

Especially at end of life, patients may request treatments whose usefulness is doubtful. For instance, a person in the end stages of chronic obstructive pulmonary disease may request that, as the disease progresses, CPR be administered each time respiration stops even when it has no chance of doing more than extending life a few hours or days in an unconscious state. It is common for such a situation to be portrayed in terms of a conflict between autonomy, on the one hand, and beneficence and the responsible use of resources on the other. (Beneficence, or nonmaleficence, is a factor because performing CPR or other procedures when they are futile can amount to brutalizing the patient.) However, futile procedures by definition do not support the patient's practical identities, and therefore requests for them are not expressions of true patient autonomy. Autonomy is about the overall arc of patient actions and abilities, and futile procedures do not work to continue that arc. In the context of agreed-upon goals, we can understand a request for treatment that is clearly futile as a case of the patient not appreciating the relevant facts.[13]

Changing Persons

Buchanan and Brock (1989) noted "several morally significant asymmetries between the contemporaneous choice of a competent individual and the issuance of an advance directive to cover future decisions"[14] (152–153). These are entailed by the following facts: (1) prognosis and treatment options may change between the time that a well-informed individual issues an advance directive and when it has to be implemented; (2) an individual's best interests may change "in radical and unforeseen ways" through time, especially in the case of illness; (3) the usual "informal safeguards" against imprudent decisions (such as family members raising objections) cannot be mobilized when advance directives are being implemented; and (4) advance directives commonly address a limited range of situations, and are silent when an actual situation arises that is different from the ones anticipated (Buchanan and Brock 1989, 153). Advance directives constructed along the lines of a Values History, emphasizing persons' practical identities and goals, eschew asymmetries (1) and (4), and are likely to mitigate the effects of asymmetry (3). Asymmetry (2) remains a difficulty.

In this section I address asymmetry (2). A radical version of it has attracted particular attention in the philosophical literature: the issue of personal identity:

Advance directives only have moral authority if the person who issued the directive and the person to whom the directive would be applied are the same person; but the very circumstances which would bring an advance directive into play are often those in which one of the necessary conditions for personal identity is not present. (Buchanan and Brock 1989, 155)

Here we are dealing with the philosophical concept in which what is at issue is whether the person who issued the directive is *the same individual person as* the person to whom the directive would be applied.

Those not familiar with the philosophical discussions of personal identity may find an example helpful. Consider a young woman, call her Constance. Constance had recently begun her undergraduate studies when she contracted meningitis and fell into a coma. The woman who awoke from the coma had Constance's body, and seemed to have Constance's knowledge, but was somewhat different in personality. Her undergraduate institution decided that the decision to admit her should be reviewed, and requested a new application and interview. They did not consider their decision to admit precoma Constance as committing them to educating postcoma Constance. We might speculate that, had they put their decision in metaphysical terms, they may have said that they were unsure that the woman who emerged from the coma was the same person as the one they had admitted to the college.

Buchanan and Brock saw two separate challenges to the authority of advance directives: first, the challenge of asymmetry (2), of applying an advance directive to the same person who now has different interests; and second, the challenge that arises when the organism corresponding to the person drafting the directive has come to correspond to a different person. Personal identity can be thought of in various ways, ranging from the view that identity of persons is the same as or dependent on the identity of their bodies, to the view that psychological continuity is sufficient for personal identity even in the case of psychological transfer to a completely new body or away from any body at all. For our discussion of advance directives, we are not as interested in cases of change of body or disembodied persons as we are in psychological change that may be great enough to constitute a change of person. The other sorts of changes considered by several authors are too far from what HCPs are likely to encounter to be of interest here (see Parfit 1984; Unger 1990).

The difference between changing interests and changing persons can be seen as a difference in degree (perhaps one in which a difference in degree can be great enough to constitute a difference in kind). The difference is in psychological profile, in personality, character, and values. These differences will presumably result in differences in goals and practical identities.[15] Presumably, one could change many personality traits with very little change in goals and practical identities. For instance, one could become more irascible, less patient, and less inclined to laughter while retaining one's other features. I suggest that these kinds of changes would not be sufficient for change of person. I suggest also that changes sufficient for change in personal identity would involve changes in goals and practical identities.

Buchanan and Brock accepted Parfit's general idea that identity of person over time can be a matter of degree (based roughly on psychological continuity). They proffered what they called a compromise position, in which advance directives bear full authority if the degree of continuity is above a certain threshold, and limited authority if below.[16]

Dresser (1989) also took questions of personal identity seriously.[17] She cited cases of "Ulysses contracts" such as occur with the psychiatry patient who checks himself in and agrees that the hospital should not let him leave for a specified period even if he begs to go, and the patient (perhaps a dialysand) who requests withdrawal of a life-saving treatment with the provision that later requests to reinstitute treatment be denied. She observed that:

... even if illness destroys a person's capacity for self-determination, the patient retains an interest in his or her present and future well-being that can conflict with the former self's preferences contained in an instruction directive. (Dresser 1989, 161)

Individuals who are incompetent to make medical decisions can still have interests, conceivable in terms of goals and practical identities, that bear weight in medical decision making. If illness has not only caused incompetence but has also caused the ill person to be a different individual person from the one who, before illness, completed an advance directive, we have good reason to doubt that the advance directive should be taken as authoritative. Again, the case in which identity of person ceases to hold can be considered as an extreme version of the case in which an individual's goals and identities have changed to a lesser degree.

What are we to do in such situations? Dresser considered ways to balance "the patient's contemporaneous interests" with "the past-expressed preferences embodied in advance directives" (165). For instance, ". . . the policy could entail focusing on the patient's present interests, unless they are too difficult to ascertain" (165). But just what are we ascertaining when we ascertain the patient's present interests? Stated preferences? Goals qua organism or qua person? The closest idea we have examined might be that of the patient's objectified subjective interest—what the patient would want to want if she were ideally rational and informed, and maintained her practical identities (or a consistent subset of them chosen from among the strongest or most central). Applying this notion allows us to respect Ulysses contracts, which are meant to ensure respect for the individual's second-order preferences, what the individual wants to want rather than what the individual actually wants at a particular time. There is a difference between having an occurrent want for A, and A being something that promotes one's goals and practical identities.

But what if the patient's objectified subjective interest changes? We are not, of course, interested in the trivial changes that come about with changes in circumstance. (One's objectified subjective interest in having a picnic with one's family may change with the weather, for example.) Rather, we are interested in changes in patterns of objectified subjective interest that come with changes in practical identities. Some events can be expected to change a person's practical identities. Religious conversion, marriage, and becoming a parent are among these. Illness may be another.

Given our account of autonomy as consistency, change in practical identity will at first be suspicious. Choices that do not fit in the arc established by the person's previous choices will seem not to be autonomous. Any number of things may be going on in such a case. The choice could flow from the adoption of a new practical identity, the agent may be acting on misinformation, the choice may have been made under coercion, or the choice may be in some other sense mistaken or accidental. When a patient claims to have changed practical identities, this claim must be assessed much as we assess the legitimacy of goals and identities in general (see discussion of "problems with goals" in chapter 2). That is, we look for consistency among the goals and identities, and between these and facts about the world.

Legitimate goal changes should be respected. This does not mean that we are giving up on the claim that autonomy requires consistency, but the consistency requirement is *provisional*. Practical identities commit us to act according to rules, but only for as long as a person maintains that identity. However, as I noted in chapter 5, there are limits to how often one can change practical identities. Adopting a practical identity is like adopting a direction for travel; if you change too often you will not succeed in going anywhere.

A significant difference exists between asserting a preference or making a request and changing one's practical identities. The latter is more robust, requires at least minimal consistency with facts and other practical identities, and commits one to other preferences in a way that a simple preference assertion does not. Preference assertions and individual requests by a patient whose care is being guided by an advance directive should not be allowed to override the provision of the advance directive. Ulysses contracts are intended to address just such concerns.

Assertion of new practical identities, on the other hand, may invalidate an advance directive that is inconsistent with the new identities and goals. We can hope that in such cases the individual thinks to make changes in the physical document and to discuss these changes with those who might be in a position to shape care. If new practical identities can invalidate advance directives in cases in which the changes are not radical enough to constitute a change in personal identity, a fortiori, they can do so in cases where the changes are radical enough.

The ability to adopt a practical identity, to commit to acting consistently in a way that coheres with one's overall circumstance, may be the best we can do as a way to understand what it means for a patient to make competent choices. Advance directives are intended to guide medical decisions when the individual becomes incompetent. The patient who is in the process of adjusting his practical identities is necessarily competent and thus should not at the same time have his medical care guided by an advance directive.

We might still worry about possible cases in which old practical identities simply do not apply to the incompetent patient. The professional basketball player whose automobile accident has left her permanently blind and temporarily in a coma is a fairly straightforward example. No medical intervention will count as promoting her identity as a professional basketball player. If this identity had been a central and structuring part of her identity, its place in her life will have to be revised to fit her new situation. We can still consider her objectified subjective interest, however, and use that to guide decisions on her behalf while she remains unable to decide for herself. The question to be considered is, what would she want to want given her practical identities, *taken in the context of her present situation?* Admittedly, this is a question we may not be able to answer. A virtue of my treatment is the fallback approach of promoting health of the patient qua organism.

Abuses

Understanding the HCP's duty in this way opens the door to abuse by those who misunderstand the patient's goals and practical identities. It would be easy to conclude that an expressed choice need not be respected because it would not be the most efficient way to pursue the patient's goals. Competent patients must be allowed to find their own ways to play out their plans, to make their own mistakes. On the other hand, if a mistake is too big the patient will no longer seem competent. Therein lies the messy part: what counts as too big a mistake? But we apply our judgment on such matters all the time. The difference between competence and incompetence is a matter of degree, not a matter of kind, and we must muddle on as best we can. We intervene with patients, as with friends, relatives, and children, when the degree is great and much is at stake. Again, transparency of reasoning can help the patient appreciate a parentalist decision based on supporting reasons. The same standard can be sought from patients when they make choices that seem irrational.

Death with Dignity

In some circumstances it is appropriate and permissible for a patient to refuse a course of action that would prolong life. A patient with a progressive and debilitating condition such as MS, ALS, or chronic obstructive pulmonary disease may have a strong preference not to continue living when mental and physical functioning become minimal. Can death be healthy for this patient when the disease progresses past a certain point? It seems like an absurd question. Indeed, Bloomfield's (2001) explanation of moral realism relies on the claim that healthy and dead are at opposite ends of the health spectrum. Whereas dying will always decrease the health of the patient qua organism, hastening death could improve health qua person. The answer must be that, whereas being dead is far from being healthy, it may be closer to health for some patients qua persons than any living state.

Reliability of Advance Directives

Several studies concluded that advance directives are not appropriate guides for medical care because of evidence that patient preferences are unstable and that patients and their proxies tend to interpret preferences differently. Thus Ditto et al. (2001) claim that their study offers an "unequivocal demonstration of the ineffectiveness of both instructional ADs [advance directives] and patient-surrogate substituted judgment" (421; see also Lee et al. 1998, 260; Kohut et al. 1997, 131). Other studies drew quite the opposite conclusion, that preferences in advance directives are fairly stable and hence can be reliable sources of information relevant to appropriate care in at least some situations (Emanuel et al. 1994; Coppola et al. 2001, 431).

I speculate that much of whatever instability is present stems from the fact that the preferences asked for by standard advance directives do not connect in a clear way with other choices the patient has made and other situations the patient has faced. Putting values (goals and practical identities) at the center would make for a more reliable document because it would tap into more stable facts about the patient.

Conclusion

Margaret L. Campbell (1995) presented a case in which a specific procedure (intubation) was prohibited by a patient's advance directive, although performing it would restore the patient to an acceptable state of health and not doing so would soon be followed by the patient's death.

The question is whether the advance directive should have been invoked in this situation because, although the patient had a progressive and serious illness (chronic obstructive pulmonary disease), he was not considered "terminally or hopelessly ill"; but this assessment is accurate only if the refused procedure is given (Campbell 1995, 227). In this case, the treatment was given. The patient improved, regained consciousness, and, after the fact, approved of the decision to intubate. This shows the benefit of constructing advance directives in terms of values rather than in terms of specific procedures. Indeed, Campbell concluded by advocating advance directives that include "statements relative to the patient's goals, life plans, health care choices, and relevant scenarios for those choices . . ." (231).

Patients want their preferences to be respected, but most recognize their limitations when it comes to anticipating their medical needs and understanding complex medical procedures and risks. Advance directives that identify goals and practical identities allow people to express themselves in a way that really reflects who they are and what they value. Moving to a model constructed on the basis of practical identities is thus likely to increase patient comfort with these documents, and hence increase the number of patients adopting them. Remember, however, that honoring autonomy does not guarantee that what the autonomous individual chooses is permissible.

We have seen that the idea of a goals-driven advance directive is not new. The AMA, Doukas and McCullough, and others[18] advocated putting values and goals at the center of our thinking about appropriate care for patients who are unable to decide on their own behalf. The ethical legitimacy, even obligation, of advance directives has been understood in terms of respect for patient autonomy. However, when we accept that the patient's values and goals determine what constitutes health for the patient qua person, we see that these documents can have grounding not just ethically but also medically. Based in practical identities and goals, they can help HCPs determine what is medically appropriate for a given patient. This is a good deal more than merely indicating what the patient would choose.

7

Talking to Patients, Training Physicians

Chapter 6 discussed implementing our theory of health in the context of end-of-life issues. Medical ethics is not just about sex and death, however. Despite the tendency among many to think that ethics is relevant only to cases that are obviously problematic, even political, every medical encounter has an ethical component.

Some contend that the ethical component in medicine has risen to prominence due to the fact that we can now cure or avoid many of the life-and-death complaints that physicians used to face, such as polio, scarlet fever, and other infections. It is rarely questioned whether administering polio vaccine is consistent with the goals of the individual (or of society, for that matter). By contrast, many medical interventions that now grab our attention seem somehow optional, their value less clear and more open to debate.[1] For instance, should insurers pay for prescriptions to reverse male-pattern baldness? If so, should they encourage all of their balding male patients to take medication for this condition? In the present medical environment it is more important than ever for HCPs to appreciate each patient's goals.

At the same time, the revolutionary advances in medical science have pushed physicians away from considering their patients as persons rather than organisms. The trend seems to be away from treating a "patient-as-person" and toward treating a "patient-as-a-bodily-machine," and even a "patient-as-a-mental-machine" (Fulford 1989). Reconceiving the patient in this way institutes a new model of the patient-doctor relationship:

Such a model is appropriate enough up to a point for scientific research; it is appropriate, too, for the relationship between the doctor and the patient's body.

. . . But it is wholly inappropriate for the relationship between the doctor and his or her actual patient. (Fulford 1989, 251–252)

The relationship between research and teaching at academic medical centers along with the perception that academic hospitals offer better care than other medical centers reinforce this tendency. It is further reinforced by the prominence of evidence-based medicine and treatment guidelines provided by HMOs and other institutions involved in regulating health care.

As we move on with this discussion of clinical connections, we must recognize that it is rare for individual clinical interactions to be explicitly determined by theories of health and disease. Instead, clinical medicine is ". . . defined and discovered principally by the resolution of individual doctor-patient accommodations" (Siegler 1981, 643).

This chapter addresses the relationship between patient and health care professional (HCP) generally in the context of the foregoing discussions. How can the understanding of health and autonomy developed in previous chapters help us to think about this relationship? What light does it shed on available models of the patient-doctor relationship? After considering these questions, we will turn to how our results stand in relation to what medical students are taught, judged from textbooks that introduce doctors-in-training to clinical work. All along, we will keep in mind our understanding of medical beneficence as developed earlier.

The Patient-Professional Relationship

Much has been said about the doctor-patient relationship.[2] Several models have been described to characterize what does and what should happen in clinical encounters. Any number of aims are possible in a meeting between a patient and an HCP. Some of them will be ethical, some economic, and so on. I am interested in identifying what type of interaction is most likely to promote health of patients qua persons. Promoting health is the characteristically medical aim of the clinical encounter. As I proposed, this aim has an ethical aspect insofar as it relates to a duty of medical beneficence, and promoting health of individuals qua persons is primary in this duty.

Although most of the discussion centers on the relationship between patients and physicians, I want to continue to think broadly about the role of HCPs, including psychotherapists, nurse practitioners, and others. That said, the primary care physician is the HCP most often in a position to choose how to relate to patients from among a variety of viable options. As the gate-keeper for patients whose insurance requires referrals before they can receive specialist care, and as the generalist to whom patients turn for everyday care, that physician is in a position to shape the health care received by patients more than any other HCP.

Among physicians, it is the primary care physician whose relationship style is most central to the provision of care (Brody 1992). Noting that the surgeon depends on a scalpel and the gastroenterologist on an endoscope, Brody suggested that the primary care physician's most significant tool is the relationship with the individual patient:

This physician can decide which symptoms are minor and which are major, when to reassure the patient, when to admit him to the hospital, when to refer him to a specialist, and when to call in a psychologist, not by cutting or peering into the body but by having the personal experience necessary to place what has changed into the context of the patient's life history and immediate environment. (Brody 1992, 58)

A competent psychotherapist will be able to do much of this, and is even more likely than the primary care physician to have the kind of relationship envisioned here. However, it is characteristic of the primary care physician to be able to identify and recommend treatment for conditions ranging from those that are characterized by psychological terms to those that are primarily physical.

The importance of the doctor-patient relationship is reflected in the way patients talk about their HCPs. According to one physician, it is common for patients to distinguish between doctors who are merely consulted or who merely show up at the bedside and those with whom they have an established relationship. In her experience, when she asks a patient, "Who is your doctor?," the answer will be an HCP with whom the patient feels a connection, even if that is not the patient's primary caregiver. She has found that patients refer to "my cardiologist" or "the cardiologist" depending on whether a relationship has been established. Thinking in this way, we would likely find a great many patients treated by doctors but "having" no doctor at all.

Robert M. Veatch (1972) described four models of the doctor-patient relationship. Under (1) the priestly model, the physician takes authority for healing the patient or for instructing the patient on what to do. This is commonly called the paternalistic model. In (2) the collegial model, the clinical encounter is more like a conversation among equals. The engineering model (3) has the physician figuring out what to do to solve a biological puzzle, generally how to return the patient's body to working order. Veatch advocated what he called (4) the contractual model. This model assigns rights and responsibilities to both the HCP and the patient, which is an equalizing factor, promoting patient autonomy in a situation of power imbalance. Contractual considerations are important, but none of these models highlights the aspect of the patient-doctor relationship we are interested in here.

A different quartet of models consists of the paternalistic (priestly), informative (alternatively called the consumer, or advisor model, and related to the scientific-engineering model), interpretive, and deliberative models (Emanuel and Emanuel 1992). "The paternalistic model assumes that there are shared objective criteria for determining what is best." This would explain why, in this model, ". . . the physician can discern what is in the patient's best interest with limited patient participation" (2221). This feature of the paternalistic model makes it most appropriate when the goal is to promote health of the patient qua organism. It will be much less effective as a way to promote health qua person, because the HCP does not have direct access to the patient's personal goals and practical identities.

In the informative model, the HCP provides the patient with information about his or her physical state and available interventions, and leaves the patient to make his or her decision as to what is appropriate. This may seem to maximize patient autonomy in that the patient is the one who makes the decisions, informed and free from coercion or interference. However, "The informative model's conception of autonomy is incompatible with a vision of autonomy that incorporates second-order desires" (Emanuel and Emanuel 1992, 2224). The physician does not step in to counter weakness of will or other complications that can put patients off the track they have chosen or want to choose for themselves. The sense of autonomy promoted by this model is thus a rather thin one.[3]

Even so, it is generally thought that American medical practice has moved from a predominantly paternalistic model toward a predominantly informative one, as autonomy has become the primary value.

Consider next the interpretive model:

The aim of the physician-patient interaction is to elucidate the patient's values and what he or she actually wants, and to help the patient select the available medical interventions that realize these values. (Emanuel and Emanuel 1992, 2221)

This model puts the physician in the role of a counselor, ". . . analogous to a cabinet minister's advisory role to a head of state." The physician supplies information, helps to clarify values, and suggests ways to implement these values (2222).

The interpretive model is the relationship most likely to promote health of the patient qua person. Patients often have to clarify what they want in their lives before they can make choices about medical care. Sometimes this means uncovering existing goals and identities, sometimes it involves increasing appreciation of how existing goals cohere with facts, and sometimes it involves forming brand new choices and preferences in the face of a decision that simply does not connect with those previously faced. All of this is necessary in order to move forward with confidence that a medical choice is consistent with medical beneficence with respect to health of the patient qua person.

The Emanuels have reservations about the possibility and appropriateness of implementing the interpretive model. They worry that it is unreasonable to expect physicians to develop skills necessary for this type of relationship. They are also concerned about physicians' ability to interpret patient values in a neutral way. Few physicians receive training to help them implement the interpretive model responsibly, and nearly all practice under strict time limitations. Those whose own values influence their effort to interpret the patient's preferences and situation may very easily sway the patient's views. The Emanuels express concern that the interpretive model too easily turns paternalistic (2224). We will return to these concerns after considering the Emanuels' fourth model.

The deliberative model involves limited advocacy by the physician. "The aim of the physician-patient interaction is to help the patient determine and choose the best health-related values that can be realized in the clinical situation . . ." (Emanuel and Emanuel 1992, 2222). The discussion is limited to health-related matters, and includes recommendations by the HCP regarding which outcomes are to be valued. Health-related values ". . . affect or are affected by the patient's disease and treatments . . ." (2222).

The HCP's role as an advocate for health-related values would seem appropriate given the HCP's status as a professional and hence as an expert on health matters. We have seen, however, that whereas HCPs have the status of experts on health qua organism, what counts as health related varies greatly when we are considering health of patients qua persons. The Emanuels are right to note that ". . . many elements of morality are unrelated to the patient's disease or treatment and beyond the scope of their professional relationship" (1992, 2222). However, as we have seen, HCPs cannot determine what counts as health related for individual patients qua persons without considering patients' specific values, and identifying these values sometimes takes work. The moral values that the Emanuels want left out often concern whether a patient's given identity or goal ought to be health related. We cannot assume that physicians have insight appropriate for advocating life plans, practical identities, and the like. Thus if we insist that they have special access to facts about which matters are health related, we must limit our understanding of what counts as such matters to issues concerning health of patients qua organisms.[4]

According to the Emanuels, the deliberative model is the best of the four. Among its virtues, they see it as promoting a workable ideal of autonomy, as cohering with our understanding of the physician's role as a caring advocate, and as avoiding paternalism (2225–26). Given the Richman–Budson concept of health of persons, however, we see that this model is too limiting.

The interpretive model is not limited in this way. It requires that the HCP listen, consider, and reflect the patient's goals and values. Thus it supports what Brody and others called "patient-centered primary care." Brody summed up patient-centered care as follows: ". . . *the primary care physician's approach to the patient's problem is grounded in the way the patient himself defines the problem*" (1992, 58–59). Patient-centered primary care promotes autonomy throughout the medical relationship by setting up a situation in which the HCP sees and conceives of the patient's complaint through the patient's own eyes (Brody 1992, 60). Not only is the treatment decision in the hands of the patient, so too is the very definition of the problem. This is the approach sanctioned by the concept of health of patients qua persons, and of the models examined so far, the interpretive model of the patient-HCP relationship comes closest to supporting it.

Like the Emanuels, I want to treat models of patient-HCP relationship as regulative ideals. It is no objection if a model has never been or cannot be fully realized. In advocating one type of relationship, I am endorsing this as something to aim for, asymptotically, under appropriate conditions. Conditions are most appropriate for using the interpretive model as a regulative ideal when an HCP is working with a competent patient with whom he or she will interact over many visits, and whose complaints are not extremely urgent. Of course, once the relationship has been established, the interpretive approach can be applied with increasing efficiency. Where patients require urgent care from a physician they have never met before, as is typical in emergency rooms, the relationship appropriately and of necessity takes on a different character.

The interpretive model is most compatible with the goal of promoting health of patients qua persons. However, it comes with very high expectations for HCPs, primary care physicians in particular. Can we expect HCPs to develop skills to facilitate the process that patients must sometimes go through as they clarify their goals? Can we expect them to apply such skills without influencing patients toward their own values? Furthermore, can we expect patients to embrace a medical encounter that includes this kind of "goal therapy"?

HCPs already have a great deal on their agendas in the current health care environment. Not only must they keep up with the latest studies and methods, they must supervise office staff, handle insurance and billing issues, and deal with pharmaceutical representatives. In this context, sensitive facilitation of goal therapy may seem like an outrageous additional burden. Even so, this is what it takes to ensure that patients are treated as persons and not just bodies. It must be done if we are to work toward improving health of patients qua persons.

One way to do this is to move some of the work to a professional or paraprofessional patient advocate. Such a person could help patients begin the process of articulating what they want from the encounter with the physician. Although this cannot replace interaction with the individual who actually provides the treatment, it can prime the pump, so to speak, and make the provision of care more efficient while still allowing for clarification of patient values that may be necessary for choosing among treatment options.

What about maintaining objectivity? The HCP is likely to have opinions about the relative value of various functions. Furthermore, given their training in the biosciences, physicians are likely to advocate health qua organism when that competes with health qua person. It is acceptable for them to have these views, but unacceptable for them to exert coercion in a way that interferes with patient autonomy.

The patient-HCP relationship involves an inherent power difference, so that the patient is easily influenced. The patient may adopt the HCP's preference in an effort to procure quality care, or may simply take the HCP's views as authoritative, and in so doing may or may not be aware of these influences. Thus HCPs must solicit and pay attention to patient preferences without influencing them. Once these preferences are on the table, however, it has to be permissible for HCPs to offer input. Indeed, it can be obligatory for them to advise the patient when, in their view, the patient is making an inappropriate choice. (Obviously, such advising, which we might call *advocacy*, has to be sensitive to cultural factors.)

Will patients stand for this? People, particularly in the United States, value the ability to get the care they want when they want it. Pharmaceutical companies have exploited this by marketing directly to consumers, many of whom feel little or no compunction about requesting prescriptions for specific drugs before any discussion with their physician. But patients also want attention. They want to be treated as persons whose identities, choices, and values are taken seriously. The interpretive model promotes that.

This constellation of concepts—health qua person and patient-centered care in the context of an interpretive model of the patient-HCP relationship—supports the gate-keeper model of a primary care physician. The gate-keeper helps guide patients to appropriate specialists, interpreting each patient's situation in a way that allows the patient to make the best use of available resources. Of course, other interests can often intervene, but at its best, this model promotes a continuing relationship with one HCP who thereby has the opportunity to do well at promoting health of the patient qua person.

Patient-Provider Communication

Communication styles employed by HCPs establish their relationship with individual patients. Studies show that communication styles can have a measurable effect on both patient satisfaction (Ong et al. 1995; Bertakis, Roter, and Putnam 1991; Putnam et al. 1985) and health outcomes (Kaplan, Greenfield, and Ware 1989; Greenfield, Kaplan, and Ware 1985). There seems to be "a correlation between effective physician-patient communication and improved patient health outcomes" (Stewart 1995, 1423).

In a review of related studies, Moira A. Stewart observed that patients are more likely to recover when physicians ask about their concerns, emotions, and expectations, and about how they understand their health problems (Stewart 1995, 1428). Good outcomes are also correlated with interventions in which the patient is able to express feelings, opinions, and information fully and "perceives that a full discussion of the problem has taken place" (Stewart 1995, 1428).[5] These data go beyond mere satisfaction with care—a patient may be satisfied even without experiencing symptom relief. Furthermore, Stewart did not include studies of psychotherapeutic relationships. The studies examined involved, for example, experience of pain after surgery and status of chronic conditions such as diabetes. Some studies were descriptive and involved little intervention in the clinical encounter. Results of descriptive, analytic studies are subject to confounding factors; it is possible that physicians who used communication techniques correlated with good outcomes shared some other feature that accounted for some or all of the difference in outcomes. However, several randomized, controlled trials reported similar results.

What is it about these communication behaviors that affects outcomes such as the experience of pain after surgery, functional status, and length of hospital stay? Emotional well-being, trust, and stress certainly play a role. Patients who "feel heard" will be less stressed and hence their bodies will be better able to heal. They are also more likely to comply with treatment (as indicated by pill counts, e.g.) (Stewart 1984).[6] We might speculate that patients who have been heard can be more confident that doctor's orders are consistent with their own goals. But we should also consider the possibility that medical outcomes improve with communication that implements patient-centered care because the patient is the one best able to determine what outcomes count as successful and patient-centered care directs attention to those outcomes.

Textbooks: What Do Medical Students Read Concerning . . .
To sort out how all this is and ought to be applied in the clinical setting, it is helpful to consider ideas that are endorsed and promoted at medical schools. Clinical education has several components. It is typical for the classroom component to decrease in importance and time commitment as a student's training progresses. In the United States, first clinical courses have titles such as "Patient-Doctor" (e.g., Harvard), "Introduction to the Patient" (e.g., Robert Wood Johnson Medical School), or simply "Introduction to Clinical Medicine" (e.g., University of California, San Diego). These are offered in the first two years of medical school, often identified as part of the preclinical curriculum.

Internet searches of medical school syllabi and reading lists revealed that several textbooks are used fairly widely in such courses. These include *Bates' Guide to Physical Examination and History Taking* (Bickley and Hoekelman 1999), *The Clinical Encounter: A Guide to the Medical Interview and Case Presentation* (Billings and Stoeckle 1989), *The Medical Interview: The Three-Function Approach* (Cole and Bird 2000), *Behavioral Medicine in Primary Care: A Practical Guide* (Feldman and Christensen 1997), *Sapira's Art and Science of Bedside Diagnosis* (Orient 2000), and *Textbook of Physical Diagnosis: History and Examination* (Swartz 1989). In the following sections we will examine what these textbooks have to say about conducting the clinical encounter and about the key components of patient-doctor communication.

The Medical Interview Considered Generally   Most aspects of patient-doctor communication fall under the general notion of the medical interview. Chapter 1 of Swartz's (1989) *Textbook of Physical Diagnosis* begins, "The main purpose of an interview is to gather all basic information pertinent to the patient's illness and the patient's adaptation to illness. An assessment of the patient's condition can then be made" (3). He later stated:

By the conclusion of the interview, the interviewer should have a clear impression of the reason(s) why the patient sought medical help, the history of the present illness, the patient's past medical history, and an understanding of the patient's social and economic position. (Swartz 1989, 9)

These are presented as the immediate goals of the medical interview. In addition, it should be recognized that the interview itself is a constituent of appropriate care. Patients sometimes need to talk and connect with a physician or other HCP. The issue of why the patient sought medical help can be useful for predicting compliance with treatment recommendations, but it can also be used to understand what aspects of life and experience the patient is concerned to preserve or restore, thereby promoting health of the patient qua person.

Cole and Bird (2000, 3) defend the "three-function approach" to the medical interview:

By using the interview as a clinical tool, the skilled physician strives to accomplish three broad objectives: (1) to establish and maintain an effective doctor-patient relationship; (2) to diagnose the patient's problems; and (3) to educate and motivate the patient to cooperate with treatment recommendations.[7]

They emphasize the three functions throughout their textbook, with key definitions in chapter 2:

The first function of the interview addresses the physician's primary task: to build and maintain an effective doctor-patient relationship. (7)

The "partnership" between patient and doctor can provide a foundation for ". . . the entire process of medical care" (7). The discussion makes clear that this "primary task" is not an end in itself, but rather a means to better outcomes, in particular the care of the patient's emotional well-being. As we have noted, research by Stewart (1984, 1995) suggests that the right sort of patient-HCP relationship can be very important in promoting satisfactory outcomes.

Cole and Bird continue:

The second function of the interview concerns the need to obtain information to assess the patient's problems. . . . The skillful physician uses data-gathering skills to assess the patient's problems and arrive at diagnostic formulations. (10)

Function 3, managing the patient's problems, gets the following treatment:

Physicians rely on the third function of the interview to educate patients and to motivate them to adhere to treatment recommendations. (11)

The authors emphasize the use of "open-ended questions," followed by more specific, targeted questions as necessary. Like the other texts examined, this one recommends reflecting (repeating, perhaps in different words) information provided by the patient as a way of eliciting more input. Of course, choosing what information to follow up on in this way, and whether to reformulate the patient's way of conveying that information introduces an element of interpretation.

Cole and Bird, as well as others, suggest "checking the patient's understanding of the problem" (Cole and Bird 2000, 38). They sometimes mean checking on whether the HCP has a good grasp of what the patient finds troubling, but more often they mean being sure that the patient understands what the HCP finds troubling.

The third function of the medical interview (developing a treatment plan) comprises seven steps:

(1) checking base-line information; (2) describing treatment goals (with options, if any) and treatment plans (with options, if any); (3) checking understanding; (4) eliciting patient preferences and commitments; (5) negotiating a plan cooperatively; (6) eliciting specific patient affirmation of intent; and (7) planning for maintenance and relapse prevention. (Cole and Bird 2000, 39)

The authors emphasize patient compliance and patient involvement in developing treatment plans, as well as getting active statements of understanding and intention. This suggests that baseline information determines the next stages with a fair degree of specificity. This is likely true for most patients.[8]

Bates' Guide to Physical Examination and History Taking presents the medical interview as a "negotiation" in which the priorities and views of the patient and the HCP are both taken into account. Note the third, fifth, and sixth elements of the following list:

The Stages of the Interview:
1. Greeting the patient and establishing rapport
2. Inviting the patient's story
3. Establishing the agenda for the interview
4. Generating and testing hypotheses about the nature of the problem(s) by expanding and clarifying the patient's story
5. Creating a shared understanding of the problem(s)
6. Negotiating a plan (includes further diagnostic evaluation, treatment, and patient education)
7. Planning for follow-up and closing the interview (Bickley and Hoekelman 1999, 6)

These authors do not advocate a strictly patient-centered view. The agenda, understanding of the problem, and plan are worked out in the context of a patient-HCP relationship that is not just about extending patient autonomy. Other interests are given voice as well.[9]

Thus the textbook literature on the medical interview encourages physicians to tap into each patient's own understanding of the situation. However, it is often unclear whether the patient's understanding is recommended as a tool for the HCP to develop an appreciation of the patient's condition as a person or only for the purpose of gathering data to formulate a diagnosis of the patient qua organism. As might be expected, patient preferences are recognized more at the point of establishing a plan for follow-up and treatment than in making a diagnosis.[10]

Obtaining the Medical History   The medical history is the centerpiece of patient-HCP communication, and can be the primary activity of a typical office visit. It is a subpart of the medical interview. What makes for a good medical history? Three themes are prominent in textbooks: asking open-ended questions, maintaining a patient-centered approach, and eliciting patient narratives.

Bates' Guide suggests:

Begin your interview with a question that allows full freedom of response, often called an *open-ended question*. "What concerns bring you here today" or "How can I help you?" After the patient answers, inquire again or even several times, "Anything else?" (Bickley and Hoekelman 1999, 7 emphasis theirs)

Other open-ended questions include, "Are there specific concerns that prompted you to schedule this appointment?" and "What made you decide to come for health care now?" (Bickley and Hoekelman 1999, 8).

Billings and Stoeckle also recommended open-ended questions, as did Orient, Cole and Bird, and Swartz. Orient made passing reference to "The patient-centered principles underlying this style of interviewing . . .", suggesting the question "Can you tell me what bothers you the most?" (Orient 2000, 17–18).[11] Another suggested question is, "Is there anything else you want to tell me?" (Orient 2000, 22). The idea is that, "In general, questions that stimulate the patient to talk freely are preferred" (Swartz 1989, 10).

Open-ended questions have several benefits. They can be more efficient than asking the patient about each possible symptom and syndrome. They also encourage sharing patient values and concerns relevant to the health care encounter:

. . . the most efficient approach is to be patient-centered, starting with eliciting the patient's complete set of concerns and questions and using open to closed cones of questions to encourage elaboration. . . . A patient-centered approach also ensures that the patient's concerns are understood and agreed on—a predictor of increased compliance. (Lipkin 1997, 1)

Whereas theorists and bioethicists emphasize the opportunity for dialogue and understanding, Lipkin sees means to efficiency and compliance.

I found it interesting that whereas Orient insists on interviewing the patient alone, *Bates' Guide* suggests asking the patient, in the presence of those accompanying her, whether she wants to be interviewed alone (Bickley and Hoekelman 1999, 6–7). This runs the risk of enabling coercion and of failing to obtain the patient's own point of view and authentic responses.

Discussions of history taking in these texts emphasize patient-centered care nearly as much as the value of open-ended questions. The first edition of the *Textbook of Physical Diagnosis: History and Examination* claimed that:

This new text focuses on the patient: his needs, his problems, his hopes. . . . Unlike many other books, this one focuses on the role of the patient as a person, *not* just a representative of a disease or a clinical state. (Swartz 1989, vi)

Ten years later, *Bates' Guide* suggested patient-centered questions as a means "To satisfy both the patient's expectations and the clinician's agenda, and to provide good health care . . ." (Bickley and Hoekelman 1999, 10).[12]

Billings and Stoeckle (1989) draw attention to the "trigger" that caused the patient to seek care, noting that ". . . the complaint itself is rarely a sufficient explanation for why this patient came in today rather than last week, next week, or never." (32) The trigger may be an important clue to the patient's values and preferences.

Another point emphasized by Billings and Stoeckle (and not missed by others) is that "Patients may have multiple problems, and the most worrisome or embarrassing ones are often saved for last" (1989, 28). Busy clinics, and there are many, that regularly depend on identifying the patient's "chief complaint" could be easily misled.

Treatment must be sensitive to individual situations, values, and roles even when they may seem straightforward. Take the case of a business executive who suffers from an injured back and arm due to a fall. Identifying the damage may be sufficient for diagnosis. But the physician should press further, to get at "the meaning of illness to this patient" (Billings and Stoeckle 1989, 42). Determining an appropriate treatment plan depends on many facts about the patient's life and goals that are independent of the specific damage to the back and arm. It depends on answers to questions such as:

How does he [the patient] ordinarily use his arm at home and at work? Will he lose his job if he cannot function normally for a few months? Is he happy to get away from work or frantic to be back? Does he have insurance, savings, pressing bills, a family to support? . . . Does he ordinarily spend his free time reading and watching television or playing tennis and working in the garden? [etc.] (Billings and Stoeckle 1989, 42)

Relevant questions will be different for patients in different demographic groups.

The language used in *Bates' Guide* harmonizes with the concept of practical identities discussed in previous chapters. The authors recommend that the clinician ask about how the patient's condition has affected daily life, with questions such as, "What can't you do now that you could do before?" They also suggest inquiring how the condition has affected the patient's abilities to function in chosen roles at work, at home, as a parent and spouse, and so on (Bickley and Hoekelman 1999, 11). Thus the textbook literature is overwhelmingly supportive of a patient-centered approach to care understood in a very general way.[13]

This discussion suggests, however, that 'patient-centered care' is used in both a weak sense and in a strong sense. In a weak sense it seeks to understand the patient's experience of the condition (one sense of 'illness') in addition to understanding the biological ground of that experience (one sense of 'disease').[14] In this weak sense, patient-centered care is important to ensure patient compliance with treatment and to administer care of the patient qua organism in a way that is respectful of the patient's preferences and personhood. The texts examined primarily support patient-centered care in this weak sense.

In contrast, the stronger sense puts the patient as person in the center of the enterprise, including defining the medical problem. Health qua person and the corollary duty of medical beneficence require patient-centered care in this sense. It is interesting that *Bates' Guide* articulates most clearly the role of the patient in creating a shared understanding and negotiated agenda for the clinical encounter. It does this while recognizing that the patient is one of several parties whose interests and preferences play a role in the provision of care.

In addition to open-ended questions and patient-centered attention, the third technique commonly recommended for obtaining the medical history is soliciting patient narratives. Obviously, these three methods are closely related and all fall under a general rubric of patient-centered techniques:

> By encouraging the patient to tell his or her own story, you not only help develop an alliance and gain a complete picture of the illness, you also obtain an overview of the issues that the patient wants to bring to your attention or feels are germane to understanding the presenting problems. (Billings and Stoeckle 1989, 18)

Patient narratives allow the patient to describe a condition in the context of everyday activities, situations, and relationships. In this way, the patient's roles, habits, and values are introduced. This can give the HCP a hook into the patient's practical identities and into understanding the ways in which the patient's condition may be interfering with autonomy.

Orient (2000) describes the history as "... the story that the physician composes to help himself and others understand the patient's disease(s) as well as the patient's illness(es)" (13). The HCP must "compose" the history using patient input. An element of interpretation must enter as the HCP works to make sense of the patient's story.

Three Ideals for Medical Encounters: Dialogue, Transparency, and Authenticity

The textbooks examined above suggest practical tools and promote patient-centered care broadly understood. However, recommended approaches are patient-centered more in the weak than in the strong sense. That is, patients' ways of understanding their conditions and experiencing their illnesses are taken into account as evidence for a medical hypothesis more than as definitive or constitutive of their condition. Building the patient-HCP relationship is often presented as a way to obtain better information, better compliance, and better outcomes rather than as a way to allow the HCP to identify with the patient and extend the patient's autonomy, or as a way to identify patient-defined problems.

Three notions can help promote productive discussions in all arenas, and can be particularly useful for promoting health qua person and patient autonomy: dialogue, transparency, and authenticity. These are ideals and may not always be fruitfully pursued. However, they support effective and ethically sound health care in the context of the relationships and techniques discussed above.

Dialogue as a means of facilitating health care goes beyond exchange of information. A patient can report symptoms, experiences, and values and listen to an HCP report a diagnosis and plan for further investigation or treatment, all without engaging in dialogue. Thus dialogue is not required for implementing the paternalist or informative (advisor or engineering) model of the clinical relationship.

Dialogue calls for careful listening and reflection, what Siegler (1981) suggested when writing of "the resolution of individual doctor-patient accommodations." These accommodations are matters of understanding, describing, and naming the patient's condition, as well as planning for possible treatment. Dialogue is the medium of mutual interpretation and meaning making, leading to what was described as "creating a shared understanding" and "negotiating a plan" (Bickley and Hoekelman 1999, 6). It requires respectful exchange in which each individual is present with personal interests and identities while making an effort to understand the other. The patient's interests and identities are certainly foremost. Furthermore, among the HCP's practical identities, the identity of member of a health care profession is the one to which the dialogue must be most attuned. Even so, dialogue requires accommodation between two individuals.[15]

The physician or other HCP does not drop out of the picture in an effort to provide patient-centered care. The HCP cannot work with the patient to understand the patient's experience of the present condition or practical identities and goals unless the patient is given some sense of how the HCP is likely to hear and react to what is being shared. In addition, the HCP is very much an agent in the provision of health care, whose own choices and autonomy are involved. Ong et al. went so far as to suggest that some aspects of the medical interview should be physician-centered. They called for integrating both patient-centered and physician-centered approaches into the medical interview so that, ". . . the patient leads in areas where he is the expert (symptoms, preferences, concerns), [and] the doctor leads in his domain of expertise (details of disease, treatment)" (Ong et al. 1995, 904).

The HCP is present not only as an expert on diseases and their treatment, but also as a person who seeks to understand and take on the interests of the patient. Thus dialogue is an important vehicle for interpretation. The patient is asked to clarify goals, and the HCP has to find in the patient's contribution some goals that he or she, charged with care of this patient, can take on.

Ganzini and Lee (1993) connected this directly to issues discussed in chapters 2 and 4:

Through empathetic discussion, the physician can assist the patient in making an autonomous decision, whereby short-term and long-term goals are not in conflict. (60)

Dialogue can also support autonomy by offering an outlet for emotions that may interfere with patient choices if not handled appropriately.[16]

Benjamin H. Levi (1999) made dialogue the centerpiece of his book, *Respecting Patient Autonomy*.

In a discussion of patient self-determination and advance directives, Lachlan Forrow (1994) held that dialogue must be accomplished in the context of an appropriately supportive relationship. After considering Dr. Seuss's book *Green Eggs and Ham*, Forrow concluded, "The fact that a patient can express a preference with utter consistency does not tell us anything about whether or not she or he understands what is at stake in the choice" (1994, S30). After all, a character in the book "unequivocally states his preference *seventy* times [Forrow's emphasis] in thirteen different scenarios" before embracing a completely opposite preference with respect to whether he will eat green eggs and ham. Forrow connected this to his point that advance care planning must be done in the context of a caring relationship between HCP and patient (S31).[17]

Although Forrow made some important points about the influence of relationships on expressions of patient preferences, he raised the specter of coercion that haunts an insistence on dialogue. Sam-I-Am's questioning in *Green Eggs and Ham*, even if well meant, borders on the belligerent and coercive. (My take on this may be related to the fact that I, like Shakespeare's Shylock and the Seuss character, have occasionally been pestered to eat ham despite a strong preference otherwise.) Dialogue is thus a delicate matter that must be implemented carefully.

Complementing dialogue is transparency. It is achieved when each party understands the reasons and reasoning behind a recommendation or action. Brody (1989) brought this ideal to bear on the issue of informed consent. He identified several standards for informed consent: (current) legal standards that invoke the notion of what a "reasonable person" would agree to, the community practice standard, the conversation standard (attributed to Jay Katz), and the transparency standard. On the transparency standard:

... "reasonably informed" consists of two features (1) the physician discloses the basis on which the proposed treatment, or alternative possible treatments, have been chosen; and (2) the patient is allowed to ask questions suggested by the disclosure of the physician's reasoning, and those questions are answered to the patient's satisfaction. (Brody 1989, 7)

Insofar as the HCP is acting on behalf of and is the agent of the patient, the patient should understand what is being done. Ideally, this understanding would go beyond the intended result. To satisfy a demand for transparency, the patient should understand the physical processes involved in the proposed treatment (or test), the hoped-for outcome, and, importantly, the HCP's reasons for choosing both this outcome and this means of achieving it. Risks of undesired outcomes are most naturally discussed in the context of why this means is recommended over other options.

Transparency in the other direction is an ideal as well. Insofar as the HCP attempts to promote the patient's identities and goals, the HCP should understand what these are and how these are related to treatment. Transparency of patient reasons and choices promotes health care that maximizes health of patients qua persons and realizes patient autonomy.[18]

The third ideal relevant to patient-HCP communication is to obtain authentic responses from the patient. Authenticity is not an easy matter. Patients feel pressure to go along with physician recommendations. Ill health can cloud judgment and make it difficult for patients to imagine or remember what it is like to be energetic or free of pain. The issue, discussed in chapter 2, of whether to give priority to a patient's preferences expressed during prescribed therapy over those expressed at other times, is also one of authenticity. Some conditions may even be primarily characterized by their tendency to impede authentic emotions, responses, and choices. Whitbeck called these "conditions of self-alienation or alienated-self conditions" (Whitbeck 1981b, 621).

Communication styles that minimize intimidation and coercion and facilitate connection and exchange are most likely to elicit authentic responses from patients.[19] Treatment based on inauthentic responses or misunderstanding of patient preferences will not promote health or autonomy.

Further Remarks on Clinical Education

The provision of health care requires sensitivity to particular circumstances and to the vast diversity of preferences and roles found even in communities that seem relatively homogeneous. Several thoughtful writers about clinical ethics and clinical practice have turned to Aristotle's discussion of virtue to describe what is involved. Some (McGee 1996; Davis 1997) identified *phronesis* (practical wisdom) as the relevant virtue. Others argued that "the clinical interaction establishes medicine as a *tekné iatrikê*, a technique of healing" (Pellegrino and Thomasma 1981, 69). *Tekné* (also transliterated "techne") is usually translated as *art*, in the sense that cabinetmaking and watch repair are arts.[20]

Developing phronesis or techne in any field requires practice over substantial periods of time. It also requires good role models and mentors (McGee 1996). Throughout this book I have argued that providing appropriate health care requires understanding patient identities, values, and goals. My point is that this requirement has grounding deeper than respect for patient dignity and identity, that it is grounded in the character of health itself. Providing health care for patients qua persons is an important part of ensuring ethically sound care. Others, as we saw in our discussion of textbooks that introduce students to clinical practice, emphasize the efficiency of techniques such as eliciting patient narratives and facilitating dialogue that allows patients to express their emotions. I emphasized how these techniques direct us to the factors that determine health of patients qua persons. We find (again) that medically good health care and ethically good health care generally converge.[21] (There are, of course, exceptions when other prima facie values conflict.)

In the face of this result, it makes sense to integrate health care ethics into a curriculum that addresses other practical issues. This is what Hope, Fulford, and Yates (1996) attempted with the Oxford Practice Skills Course that was ". . . designed to integrate training in ethics, medical law and communication skills into the curriculum. . . ." The foreword (by Caroline Miles) praised the course as a success, indicating that its main elements have become regular parts of the curriculum at Oxford "throughout the three years of the clinical course" (Hope, Fulford, and Yates 1996, vi). The seminars are nicely planned out, and offer parallel and connecting treatment of topics from perspectives of ethics, law, and communication skills. The course implements a diversity of modern teaching techniques, including multimedia and peer discussion.

But is it true that the three pillars of the clinical skills course—law, ethics, and communication skills—are integrated into the curriculum? There are three years of clinical instruction at Oxford. The Practice Skills Course is designed to use medical personnel as instructors or coinstructors throughout. But the sessions are identified as practical skills seminars, putting the topics into a sort of academic ghetto separated from the core curriculum. The first year has 24.5 hours of instruction (Hope, Fulford, and Yates 1996, 6–7). That sounds substantial. But consider that an average American graduate seminar in philosophy meets for closer to thirty-six hours in a given semester. In the second year the time committed to the Practice Skills Course drops to seven hours, in the third year to two (Hope, Fulford, and Yates 1996, 6). Thus the entire three-year course meets for less than one semester of one graduate seminar in the humanities. Admittedly, fifteen hours of this is in a tutorial setting, but the tutorial groups are six to eight students, not the one or two traditional for Oxford undergraduates. The Oxford course is clearly a wonderful start. There can be no doubt, as well, that the skills it promotes are further supported in other aspects of the clinical training experience. It does not, however, seem sufficient.

More promising are the standards for core competencies adopted by the Accreditation Council for Graduate Medical Education (ACGME). As the accrediting organization for programs in the United States that offer clinical training for graduates of medical schools (i.e., residency programs), the ACGME has begun implementing new standards based on skills rather than on core knowledge. Outcomes-based assessment, intended to measure student competency, is replacing evaluation of syllabi and instruction.

Specifically, "The residency program must require its residents to obtain competencies in . . . 6 areas . . . to the level expected of a new practitioner" (ACGME Outcome Project, 1999). The six areas are patient care, medical knowledge, practice-based learning and improvement, interpersonal and communication skills, professionalism, and systems-based practice. Individual programs are expected to develop curricula to achieve the outcomes outlined, as well as means of measuring and improving the effectiveness of these curricula. The American Society for Bioethics and Humanities (ASBH) established the Task Force on

Graduate Medical Education on Bioethics and Humanities to support programs in this effort.

The ACGME's description of professionalism is most explicitly connected to ethical concerns. Residency programs are expected to develop professionalism "as manifested through a commitment to carrying out professional responsibilities, adherence to ethical principles, and sensitivity to a diverse patient population" (ACGME Outcome Project 1999). The ASBH task force noted that the other competencies also have components that are explicitly ethical or are integral parts of the ethical provision of care (Doukas 2002). The patient care competency calls for compassionate care, the interpersonal and communication skills competency calls for ". . . effective . . . teaming with patients," and so forth.

The ACGME requirements allow that there may be many different ways to develop core competencies in new doctors. This will allow residency programs to retain their diverse traditions and cultures while meeting accreditation standards. The scheme as a whole is notable for its effort to institutionalize the notion that the practice of medicine involves skills, so that being a good HCP is a matter of having a certain type of virtue—something like practical wisdom or techne—rather than (or in addition to) a store of factual knowledge. The ACGME's presentation of these competencies, which weaves ethical concerns with technical competence and general professionalism, offers potential for true integration of ethics training into clinical training.

Conclusion

Part I of this book addressed issues in philosophy of science and presented a theory of what it is for human beings to be healthy. Our discussion of the patient-HCP relationship shows that the metaphysics of health can help guide medical care. The Richman–Budson theory of health of patients qua persons offers support for a relationship between patient and HCP that is interpretive and built through dialogue that strives for transparency and authenticity.

Care that truly supports the health of patients qua persons must be patient-centered in the strong sense. That is, it must seek not only understanding of underlying biological phenomena classified by traditional nosologies, but must uncover and respond to problems as understood by the patient. Sometimes that understanding will involve accommodation between patient and HCP, arrived at through dialogue. Thus our metaphysical conclusion is relevant to determining what counts as medically appropriate care.

The connections and mutual support between the metaphysics of health—what counts as medically appropriate care and what counts as ethically appropriate care—suggest we would do well to teach these connections to those training to be health care professionals. Learning to think of health in terms of patients qua persons provides a much richer set of reasons for patient-centered care than merely trying to achieve better pill counts.

8
Conclusion: What Every Doctor Should Know about Metaphysics

Those who have been following along since chapter 1 have traversed an ambitious range of philosophical topics. We have traipsed through the terrain of philosophy of science, explored the environs of ethical theory, and breached the borders of bioethics. It would be absurd to suggest that there is only one viable path through these wilds. I have tried to show that the path I have chosen is reasonable, and that it reflects our considered thinking about what it means for human beings to be healthy. Each path has pitfalls, and I doubt not that I have fallen into some. But the trek stops here. We have mounted to the summit. We can now look back on where we have been and glance toward adjacent territories that we did not explore on this journey.

Where We Have Been

We began by considering the subject of medicine generally, and the relationship between the biomedical sciences and physical sciences. Noting the way that biomedical sciences work with generalizations that allow exceptions and variations, it became clear that these generalizations were normative. Based on this discussion, I defended the legitimacy for biomedical science of teleological terms such as "function" and "goal-directed." I then offered a four-fold taxonomy of theories according to the roles that normativity can play. One type of theory I called "embedded instrumentalist." These theories describe an equilibrium between goals and states of affairs, where the equilibrium is what satisfies the concept. Embedded instrumentalism is different from mere instrumentalism, as one can regard the equilibrium as good in itself.

The Richman–Budson theory of health was introduced and developed in chapter 2, and can be summarized as follows: an individual *A* is in a state of health when *A* is able to reach or strive for a consistent set of goals actually aimed at by *A*. Where *A*'s goals are strongly inconsistent in ways inaccessible to *A*, the relevant set of goals is that determined by the (idealized) objectified subjective interest of *A*. *A* will be unhealthy when false beliefs are central to *A*'s most dearly held goals. When we examine *A* as a biological organism, we find a set of goals that may be incompatible with the goals *A* adopts as a conscious agent with plans for his or her life. Rather than try to adjudicate between these two sets of goals, we embrace the conclusion that there may be two answers as to whether a given state is healthy for *A*. That is, we allow that a conflict may exist between the health of *A* qua organism and the health of *A* qua person.

The Richman–Budson theory allows that what counts as healthy for a patient qua person can vary from individual to individual according to each person's goals. It can also explain how what counts as healthy can change in an individual who adopts different goals for a new stage of life (as with someone who chooses to become a parent) or for different roles in the same stage of life (as was the case for Witty Ticcy Ray).

This theory is cognitivist in that it entails that there are true and false claims about health. Of course, the truth-value of health claims about an individual will be most obvious when that individual has clear goals predicated on primarily true beliefs. This paradigm case may turn out to be rare.

At the end of chapter 2 we began to see the implications of our theory for patients and clinicians. Most obvious is the importance of talking to patients about goals. If the aim of medical care is to promote health qua person and health qua person depends on individual goals that may not be obvious to the HCP, without appropriate talk about goals, medical care runs the risk of failure. Most patients may have perfectly predictable goals. However, as I emphasized in the conclusion to chapter 2, the most competent HCP cannot know what would count as healthy for the patient qua person before gathering a great deal of information about the patient's individual concerns. This is a consequence of what it means for persons to be healthy.

We spent some time in chapter 2 considering problematic sets of goals—goals that are unrealistically high, inappropriately low, inconsistent, and so on. These discussions suggested that some problematic goals may in part be the result of maladaptive cognitions in the form of false beliefs. This in turn supports the idea that cognitive therapy, which seeks to help people experiencing various kinds of distress by applying itself directly to beliefs rather than feelings, should be available as part of regular health care for individuals with apparently unrealistic, self-defeating, or inappropriate goals.

The issue of unethical goals also arose, forcing us to consider whether such goals should count in the assessment of health qua person. There being no reason to exclude them, we recognized that health may, in particular circumstances, compete with other values. In such cases, making a patient healthy may turn out to be immoral.

The distinction between the goals of an individual qua organism and the goals of the same individual qua person can be blurry. Features valued in particular cultures (such as very small feet in women) could be biological abnormalities that help an individual to survive and reproduce in a particular environment; a condition that would otherwise be considered unhealthy may be precisely what allows a certain individual to earn a living.

The Richman–Budson theory's distinction between health qua organism and health qua person will seem to some like a distinction between health and, what is a different concept altogether, quality of life. In my exposition, the difference between the concepts comes out in the notion of richness. Health qua person is a balance between personal goals and abilities no matter what the goals may be. Quality of life assessments take into account the richness (or poverty) of an individual's goals. Like Nordenfelt's (1994b) bank clerk, an individual who is healthy with respect to a relatively poor set of goals can be as healthy as one with a richer set. Because what counts as a richer set of goals is dependent on cultural values, quality of life is further distinguished from health qua person in being culturally relative.

Having addressed problems with goals of persons, there remained the issue of what to do when health qua person and health qua organism actually conflict in an individual. Given the conclusion that both are aspects of health, we must see this as the basis of conflicting duties of medical beneficence. We sought a reason for acting on one of these duties rather than the other. For this, I invoked the Kantian notion of humans as ends in themselves. Through his notion of autonomous individuals as members of the kingdom of ends, Kant provided a framework for understanding why it is that we should value the considered choices of moral agents. This framework allows us to justify valuing the health of individuals qua persons over the health of individuals qua organisms, while at the same time explaining the normativity in embedded instrumentalist theories of health. Our Kantian understanding of the value of human preferences was developed in the context of Korsgaard's concept of a practical identity. When we understand the value of human choices in this way, the health of human organisms falls into place in the service of the autonomous choices of persons.

This way of formulating the relationship between health qua person and health qua organism has its problems, generally having to do with autonomy. I have acknowledged, if not overcome, many of these. Some are smoothed over by moving away from an emphasis on individual choices and toward packets of duties that come with practical identities.

Kantian ethics usually is accompanied by talk of duties and principles, and the discussion here is no exception. Citing Beauchamp and Childress's coherentism, I advocated checking principles against cases in the same sort of reflective equilibrium that we engaged in when, in part I, we developed our theory of health. I also maintained that the duties of medical beneficence that HCPs bear are subject to conflict with other ethical duties, including duties to promote justice, prevent harm to others, use resources wisely, and the like.

In the context of our preference-satisfaction (embedded instrumentalist) theory of health, the widely accepted view that duties of medical beneficence often conflict with respect for patient autonomy comes under scrutiny. Because promoting health qua person requires that an individual's preferences drive the goals of medical care, and these preferences are also what direct us in acting on a duty to respect autonomy, the two duties coincide. Conflicts over these duties can be understood as being between autonomy and health qua organism, or as communication problems. They could also be what we might call problems of engineering—

disagreements, misunderstandings, or apprehension about how to move the patient from the present condition to a healthier one. Parentalist concern for the health of the patient qua person falls into place similarly. Insofar as these duties involve respecting the practical identities of persons, they are also duties of respect for persons.

Part III addressed what I called clinical connections. Advance directives are intended to extend patient autonomy into situations, generally at the end of life, in which direct exercise of autonomy is not possible. However, most patients recognize that, even when at their most able, they have limited ability to make informed choices in the face of complex medical options. This is especially true when risk is involved. For this reason, I advocated moving to a model of advance directives constructed on the basis of practical identities. The Values History is one model for this.

The topic of advance directives offered further fuel for the thesis that medical choices can find at least part of their footing in the metaphysics of health. As with other practices, construction of advance directives has been understood in terms of promoting patient autonomy. However, an advance directive based in practical identities and goals not only promotes autonomy, but can also help HCPs determine what is medically appropriate for a given patient qua person.

Finally, we examined the relationship between patient and HCP. To put the Richman–Budson theory into operation requires a strongly patient-centered approach to care. Surveying an array of different models of the doctor-patient relationship, I advocated one that is interpretive and built on dialogue that strives for transparency and authenticity. We saw again in this exploration the practical implications of the metaphysical theory expounded in part I.[1]

Where We Have Not Been

Several bordering territories remain where we have not trespassed, and it is worth taking a moment to mention just a few of them. As I have noted, there is much to say about disability, autonomy, and health. Some of what I said here about personal goals, particularly in the context of rehabilitation, is relevant to disability issues, but I barely scratched the surface. In particular, I neglected the issue of those with permanent cognitive disabilities who may be unable to form preferences. I would not claim that the health qua organism of such individuals may be sacrificed in the service of the preferences of some other individual who more strictly satisfies traditional concepts of autonomy, although this may seem to follow from my account. Unfortunately, resolution of this issue will have to wait for another time.

I said much about duties of medical beneficence and respect for autonomy, but several other classes of duty are also important in the medical context. They were left aside only because they are less directly related to our theory of health. In addition to duties, values such as trust, and virtues such as *phronesis* and *techne* received little attention.

In my response to possible objections based on values associated with autonomy (in chapter 5), I proposed that the framework of practical identities allows individuals to build interconnectedness with others into their self-conception. In a very weak way, this suggests that bridges can be built between my Kantian exposition of autonomy and theories of relational autonomy, as well as the ethics of care. There may even be a trail from a preference-satisfaction concept of health to these important views that avoids Kantian concepts of autonomy altogether. Blazing that trail is a worthy project for another day.

Aside from anecdotes and scattered references to the literature, empirical work on how people apply health-related terms and how HCPs and patients actually communicate did not occupy our attention. Sociolinguists and others who trade in careful observation of human behavior and attitudes make important contributions. Our work took the more theoretical, analytic flavor of philosophy. I did not attempt the difficult but promising task of marrying the two approaches.

Philosophy is not the only humanities discipline to turn its attention to medicine. Scholars of literature have contributed a great deal by exploring the role that narrative plays in individuals' lives and how narrative can be used to develop an understanding of illness and health. The relationship between narrative and practical identities is a promising topic left unexplored.

In focusing on health, treatment, and the goals of individuals, this book pays scant attention to the larger context and units that interact in the provision of medical care. These larger units, including families, communities, institutions (including hospitals), and the medical profession itself, can have goals and interests. It is possible to talk of healthy institutions and healthy communities. Although health care is not provided to individuals in a vacuum, the "health" of these larger units was put aside in favor of topics that help us to understand health of individuals.

Further Frontiers

When philosophers of science discuss what makes for a good theory and why we might prefer one theory to another, they cite such "virtues" as simplicity, covering the data, and fruitfulness (e.g., Kuhn 1962). The Richman–Budson theory of health is not particularly simple, but I think it does a good job of covering, even explaining, the data of our intuitions concerning human health. It is certainly no slacker when it comes to fruitfulness. The previous section described several projects beyond what we have done here, and there is work to do applying the theory in other realms. For instance, our examination of medical education stopped short of looking at mentoring in clinical education beyond textbooks and classrooms. Particular areas of medicine have puzzles that could be illuminated by application of our theory. I invite the reader to join the continuing journey.

Notes

Chapter 1

1. On this topic, Mark Siegler (1981) wrote:

"At its limit, the model of disease as an objective biological state represents an analytic, scientific view in which disease and specific etiology serve as the paradigm, and in which it is argued that dysfunctional assessments involve no value judgments. In this view, sometimes referred to as the functionalist model of medicine, disease is a fact. In contrast, the extreme relativistic model of disease holds that biological derangements may not be very relevant to dysfunctional states, and that all functional assessments—both somatic and psychological—involve only value judgments" (629).

Siegler allowed that intermediate views are possible.

2. This view of science is consistent with the existence of *ideals* in the sense of idealizations. Chemists may imagine an ideal gas, physicists a perfectly elastic collision, but they do not criticize gasses for being less than ideal or collisions for being less than perfectly elastic.

3. Were we to add sufficiently detailed descriptions of the completers to the statement of the law, we might be able to state the law in such a way that there are no longer mere exceptions. The problem is, however, that much of this description would refer to types of a science more basic than that of the law in question. Thus we would no longer have a law of the science we thought we were engaged in.

4. See Fodor 1981 and 1991.

5. Seventeenth-century philosopher Nicolas Malebranche called the attribution of causal powers to ordinary objects "*The most dangerous error of the philosophy of the ancients*" (Malebranche 1997, 446). When we believe that vegetables can be the causes of tasty pleasures, he suggested, we are justifying paganism. He admonishes that ". . . one should not render sovereign honor to leeks and onions . . ." (447).

6. Robert M. Sade's Aristotelian view of health highlights several attractive features of this approach. Sade claims that there are objective facts about what

constitutes human flourishing, and that these facts are determined by the nature (and hence the function) of human beings:

". . . the virtues and good required for a flourishing life[,] are universal and objectively discoverable, but the exact weighing of these values to achieve fulfillment for a particular person is highly individualized . . ." (Sade 1995, 522).

This theory allows for variation in how we weight various goals, but claims that some components of human flourishing have intrinsic value. I do not want to make that claim. First of all, I think that we can do without it, and if we *can* do without positing something such as intrinsic value, I think we *ought* to do without it. It is worth some trouble to explore whether we are constrained to add such properties to our worldview.

A second reason for rejecting the claim that there are components of human flourishing with intrinsic value is that if we accept the components having to do with the proper working of organs such as hearts, we will end up having to let in the components having to do with the proper working of organs such as ovaries. But for many women their personal goals would best be served if their ovaries consistently failed to release eggs and thus failed to flourish. I do not see how, in a view such as Sade's, we can embrace heart virtues without embracing ovary virtues.

7. In a personal communication, one medical researcher called the tale "insulting to all modern biologists" and suggested that it represented a sort of backward thinking about science that has contributed to a decline in the relevance of philosophy to the general public.

8. Szasz also allowed that medicine makes use of teleology: "Cells, tissues, organs, and human beings *qua* biological organisms have natural functions, but human beings *qua* moral agents do not" (Szasz 2000, 3 abstract).

9. It is important to note that some X can have intrinsic value without it being the case that anyone recognizes its value. Interesting empirical studies have evaluated how much members of various demographic groups value health (see Lau, Hartman, and Ware 1986). However, empirical studies concerning whether people value health, or how much and in what ways they do so, can neither confirm nor disconfirm a theory about whether health in fact has value.

10. "The failure of some writers on the concept of health to recognize the integration of functioning that characterizes health has led them to assume that an increase in health, in any positive sense of health, would be identical with an increase in isolated abilities . . ." (Whitbeck 1981b, 618).

Chapter 2

1. Fulford's emphasis on illness as failure of action makes his theory like ours in some respects—action involves goals; failure to act is failure to reach a given goal.

2. Cf. *Nichomachean Ethics*, book VI, chapter 3.

3. Clayton's objection is discussed further in chapter 3.

4. Consider also the following description of singer-songwriter Lucinda Williams. The author portrays Williams as dependent on bouts of serious depression for her art (and hence her living):

". . . Williams's depressions are legendary; "Am I too blue for you?" is the refrain of one song devoted to them. . . . And these moments can be marked by weeping fits that go on for days. Williams now believes that the songs she writes when she has reached this therapeutic, unprotected rawness are her best; and that she has to go through this kind of trauma in order to write" (Buford 2000, 59).

5. Nordenfelt (1995) also made the claim that someone with extremely limited goals "will soon realize" that being "completely apathetic or lazy" in this way is counterproductive because it creates unhappiness (212). He needed this to be the case because of his claim that goals relevant to an assessment of health are those the satisfaction of which is required for minimal happiness.

6. Thanks are due to Michael Comer for helpful conversation on this issue.

7. These suggestions cohere with the development of cognitive therapy by Aaron T. Beck and others. The application of cognitive therapy techniques to depression in particular is discussed in *Cognitive Therapy of Depression* (Beck et al. 1979, 14–15).

8. Nordenfelt also put in this category goals that happen not to contribute to the satisfaction of long-term goals due to bad luck or other unforeseeable failure, but did not consider these to be particularly problematic for SG theories.

9. For a discussion of this issue, see Davidson 1984 and Davidson 1980 (221–22).

10. Burgess et al. (1999) raised the issue of whether this way of thinking is culture-specific:

"The most commonly cited ground for overriding religious refusals of treatments is that children must be given a chance to choose for themselves. . . ."

"Cultural and spiritual values leading to contrary values [contrary, that is, to preserving the life of the child] are only permitted influence in cases of uncertainty of outcome" (165).

11. Plato and others argued that immoral actions are always bad for the agent. Because I do not believe that these arguments show that immoral actions are bad for the *health* of the agent, I discuss immoral goals here and not in the section on counterproductive goals.

12. Whitbeck (1981b) suggested that the issue of troubling or seemingly irrational goals can be solved by seeing how they can be subordinated to other, non-troubling ones:

"The peculiar goal is only a means to some other end, and . . . if the further end were attained, the person would be satisfied and abandon the peculiar one. . . . Nothing in this argument turns on a specification of the goals that are thought to be irrational or peculiar. The point is only that if we are willing to apply the term 'irrational' to a goal, we are also inclined to say that the goal is only a means to some further end which we may regard as rational" (617).

13. Clearly the goals of the BDD patient are health related. I discuss them here because of the issue of reinterpretation and because they have an ethical dimension. The issue of BDD was brought to my attention by Sara Goering in her response to my presentation with Andrew Budson, "Health of Organisms and Health of Persons" at the Pacific Division meetings of the American Philosophical Association, Albuquerque, NM, April 2000 (2000a).

Ian Hacking suggested that some conditions such as apotemnophilia (a form of BDD) are "transient" illnesses that are in part produced by historical-societal influences and conditions. For a discussion, see Elliott 2000.

14. The principle of totality states that it is impermissible to remove parts of the body unless it is absolutely required in the interest of the body as a whole, as in cases of appendicitis or advanced gangrene.

15. I add the word "apparent" here because Stuttaford (2000) suggests that the two Falkirk patients may actually be in a biologically better situation after their amputations, since amputees are statistically more likely than others to be in long-term personal relationships. Thus perhaps surgery *is* healthy for patients with BDD who request amputations, even when considering health of the individuals qua organisms. However, the risks associated with surgery and the pre-occupations associated with BDD make me think otherwise.

16. Don Marquis (in conversation) objected to my treatment here, proposing that the reason we do not like to amputate in these cases is not merely ethical or aesthetic, but rather has to do with the fact that the effect of amputation is permanent. The patient loses the leg, which can be considered (in Rawls's terms) a "primary good," forever. Goals may change, but legs do not grow back. For a related discussion, see Buchanan et al. 2000, 80f.

17. Along these lines, Fulford offered the case of Mr. A. B. Fulford suggested that it is precisely the sort of case we should keep in mind when considering theories of health (Fulford 1989, x–xi).

18. In a discussion of happiness and quality of life, Nordenfelt (1994b, 55) stated:

". . . the non-satisfaction of a certain number of wants is compatible with complete happiness in the want-equilibrium sense. Consider the person who wants his or her life to be an adventure or a struggle, in general to be somewhat unpredictable. In more theoretical terms this may mean that this person has a higher-order want which is such that he or she does not want all first-order wants to be continuously satisfied. The person may indeed want certain problems to arise in order to remain alert and highly aware. This second order may indeed have a high priority" (55).

19. "What should be counted as a piece of obstruction or opposition, or in general what should be counted as elements of an acceptable situation is not a neutral or objective affair. This involves an ideological judgement, either made

normatively by the person who ascribes a state of health or illness to someone, or made descriptively with reference to a particular set of societal norms. . . . According to the primary use [of the phrase 'A is disabled'], . . . the speaker him or herself defines the set of accepted circumstances. . . .

"According to the secondary use, the speaker implicitly refers to some commonly accepted background—what might be called *standard* circumstances" (Nordenfelt 1995, 213).

20. For example, individuals with sickle cell trait seem to be particularly well adapted to a subset of the environments implied by the goals of the human body—those containing malaria-carrying insects.

21. Nordenfelt (1994b) described the role of the environment thus:

"While being a platform for action the environment also sets the *limits for our goals in life*. We cannot seriously want to achieve anything in every environment" (36).

22. Whitbeck (1981b) put this point well:

"Because of the importance of . . . factors that bear on a person's health and lie outside of the scope of medical expertise, decisions about the appropriateness of some medical intervention, that is, decisions about whether that intervention is likely to produce a net increase or enhancement in a person's health, cannot be decided on the basis of medical expertise alone" (625).

Chapter 3

1. I offer brief remarks on duties and goods near the start of chapter 4.

2. ". . . by 'health' we mean the experience of well-being and integrity of mind and body. It is characterized by an acceptable absence of significant malady, and consequently by a person's ability to pursue his or her vital goals and to function in ordinary social and work contexts. By this definition we aim to stress a traditional focus on bodily wholeness and general well-working, on the absence of malfunction, and on the resultant ability or capacity to act in the world" (Hastings Center 1999, 19).

3. "Although there is no inherent contradiction between care and cure, the bias toward the latter has often done harm to the former" (Hastings Center 1999, 8).

4. "On the whole, patients' choices can and should be accepted. On the other hand, people who are incapacitated by disease or trauma should not be abandoned to their autonomy, that is, merely given the 'facts' and asked to make a decision. This is a form of moral abandonment" (Pellegrino and Thomasma 1988, 17–18).

Häyry (1991) wrote similarly that:

". . . concern for the patient's right to self-determination does *not* imply that the physician should psychologically abandon the patient: a doctor who merely spreads the options in front of the patient and then says 'Go ahead and choose, it's your life' is not anti-paternalistic but negligent" (102).

5. Wulff presents his Samaritan principle as one of three principles characterizing "The ethical foundation of the public health services of the Nordic countries . . ." (Wulff 1995, 297), the others being justice and respect for autonomy.

6. The notion of a prima facie duty is, of course, borrowed from W. D. Ross. (1930, chapter 2). For a quick primer on this concept, see Munson 2000, 17–18.

7. Readers will note the similarity between my approach and that taken by Beauchamp and Childress (2001).

8. Ignoring, of course, issues of whether this could really be the same individual person.

9. Ostenfeld (1994) provides a discussion of the Aristotelian notion of quality of life. We discussed Aristotelian concepts of health briefly in chapter 2.

10. Several other theorists have also seen a central role for individual preferences. See Hare 1981; Brandt 1979; and Parfit 1984, esp. 493–502.

11. "Health economists often emphasize that, in the name of efficiency and equity, scientific measurements of the quality and quantity factors of life and health should be employed, so as to facilitate decisions concerning resource allocation. But as the term 'scientific' in the context of modern medicine and health care is mostly taken to refer to the exact and objective *natural sciences*, quality-of-life studies have since their advent in the 1940s mostly been based on the 'objective' requirements of reproducibility and measurability by external observation. The problem with these requirements . . . is that they may . . . produce quite unreliable results" (Häyry 1991, 103–04).

12. "In order for P to be at least minimally happy, then all those conditions which have a high priority for P, in an absolute sense of the word, must be materialized. Where this line goes in any concrete sense must vary much between different people. People have different temperaments and traits of character. The impatient and spoilt person is such that he or she becomes unhappy for the most trivial reasons. To such a person then almost every want has a high priority. The patient or stoic person, on the other hand, is such that he or she can meet most adversities without falling below the level. To this person very few matters in life have a high priority" (Nordenfelt 1994b, 51).

13. "As long as a person still has an unactualized set of potential wants he or she can become happier in the richness sense of the word" (Nordenfelt 1994b, 53).

14. Sandøe and Kappel (1994) stated that no comparison can be made between two situations such as those of young P and older P on the basis that quality of life is judged by sets of values that are incommensurable.

15. Cf. Swanson et al. 1999. This example was brought to my attention by Andrew Budson.

Chapter 4

1. Bruce Miller identifies "three elements of the capacity for autonomy (agency, independence, and rationality)" (Miller 1995, 217) corresponding to Beauchamp and Childress's elements of intention, absence of outside control, and understanding.

2. "To restrict adequate decision-making by patients and research subjects to the ideal of fully or completely autonomous decision-making strips their acts of any meaningful place in the practical world, where people's actions are rarely, if ever, fully autonomous" (Beauchamp and Childress 2001, 59).

3. R. M. Hare (1981, 108) took this idea even a step further, stating that universalizability is implied in the very meaning of moral language.

4. ". . . we are interested above all else in a number of apparently simple deductive problems which so many intelligent people almost invariably got wrong" (Wason and Johnson-Laird 1972, 2).

5. An example of the gambler's fallacy is the person who tosses a coin for the eleventh time, and judges from the fact that the first ten came up heads that the likelihood that the eleventh one will come up tails is better than 50-50.

6. Stich's interest is to show that folk psychology does not provide an accurate model of how human minds actually work, and that therefore philosophical theories of mind that use folk psychology as their model for human cognition, including those of Daniel Dennett (1987, 1991) and Donald Davidson (1980), are misguided.

7. "Since, as feminists and others have pointed out, agents are socially embedded and seem to be at least partially constituted by the social relations in which they stand, if attributing autonomy to agents is indeed to presuppose individualism or atomism, then it seems that the attempt to articulate autonomy rests on a mistake" (Mackenzie and Stoljar 2000, 7).

8. According to the Foucauldian, "Agency must be reconceptualized not as a matter of individual will but as an effect of the complex and shifting configurations of power" (Mackenzie and Stoljar 2000, 10–11).

9. ". . . diversity critiques parallel postmodernist critiques in challenging the assumption that agents are cohesive and unified. Such critiques claim that each individual has a 'multiple identity,' which reflects the multiple groups to which the individual belongs" (Mackenzie and Stoljar 2000, 11).

10. Consider the following definition of 'patient' offered by the Oxford English Dictionary (2001):

"A person or thing that undergoes some action, or to whom or which something is done; 'that which receives impressions from external agents' . . . correlative to agent, and distinguished from instrument; a recipient."

11. ". . . no choice is rational which violates the status of rational nature as an end: rational nature becomes a limiting condition of the rationality of choice and

action. It is an unconditional end, so you can never act against it without contradiction. If you overturn the *source* of the goodness of your end, neither your end nor the action which aims at it can possibly be good, and your action will not be fully rational" (Korsgaard 1996a, 123).

12. "Only a rational being has the capacity of acting according to the conception of laws, i.e., according to principles. This capacity is will. Since reason is required for the derivation of actions from laws, will is nothing else than practical reason" (Kant 1959, 29).

13. "But the distinctive feature of humanity, *as such*, is simply the capacity to take a rational interest in something: to decide, under the influence of reason, that something is desirable, that it is worthy of pursuit or realization, that it is to be deemed important or valuable, not because it contributes to survival or instinctual satisfaction, but as an end—for its own sake. It is this capacity that the Formula of Humanity commands us never to treat as a mere means, but always as an end in itself" (Korsgaard 1996a, 114).

14. "Conceptions of our practical identity are typically contingent, and often come about without any choice on our part, as Korsgaard notes. I happen to be the daughter of certain parents, the mother of a particular child, a certain person's neighbor, even a fan of Gilbert and Sullivan, all through no choice of my own. These things are not and never have been up to me in the way that some practical identities are (being married, for example). And many of these things could have been otherwise. I could have produced a different child, had a different neighbor, hated light opera" (Cohon 2000, 68).

15. ". . . on Korsgaard's view I take an impulse to be a reason for me to act, and I make it my reason to act, when, on reflection, I endorse it. First I identify with it, which is, at least in part, finding it to be connected in the right way with one or more of my practical identities. In endorsing the consideration as a reason, however, I also make a law for myself to act in this way. The normativity I thus impart to my impulse is imposed by my will, in that I give myself this maxim as a law. . . . Desires, then, are not automatically normative for me. I make some of them normative by means of my practical identification and self-legislation. The others are not reasons" (Cohon 2000, 66).

16. A further pair of personal examples suggests itself. When I was an undergraduate at Haverford College, someone seen committing a minor moral indiscretion (such as cutting to the front of the lunch line) was likely to be greeted with a cry of "Remember your Quaker principles!" Similar behavior at Wadham College, Oxford, during that period was met with "Remember your socialist principles!" Clearly membership in those academic communities brought with it the presumption of distinct moral identities.

17. "What brings 'objectivity' to the realm of values is not that certain things *have* objective value, but rather that there are constraints on rational choice" (Korsgaard 1996a, x).

18. "Many autonomous actions could not occur without others' material cooperation in making options available. Respect for autonomy obligates profes-

sionals in health care and research involving human subjects to disclose information, to probe for and ensure understanding and voluntariness, and to foster adequate decision-making" (Beauchamp and Childress 2001, 64).

19. "... paternalism should be understood to mean a medical decision to benefit a patient without full consent of the latter" (Pellegrino and Thomasma 1988, 10).

20. Dominic Sisti shared helpful conversation on cases of this sort.

21. I am aware of some important objections to this way of presenting things. See chapter 8.

22. Note how this exposition coheres with a commonsense notion of autonomy, described by physician Dennis H. Novack as "... the ability to act from a stable sense of self and values without needing the approval of others to do what is right" (Cole and Bird 2000, 245).

Chapter 5

1. Cf. Patricia J. Williams's (1991) "mythodology" of critical legal studies, especially the parable before the first chapter.

2. Judith Wilson Ross (1998) raised different issues regarding the "practice guidelines" generated from outcomes research.

3. "The identification of those patterns of functional achievement that are most feasible or likely and those that are most valuable requires different tactics. The sequence through which individuals would choose to recover activities, if that choice were under their control, is not necessarily the same as the most probable patterns of recovery" (Stineman 2001, 152–53).

4. Principlism has sometimes been said to offer competing, incommensurable values. For instance, autonomy and beneficence have been treated as competing. We have shown how at least these two can be made commensurable in the realm of health of individuals qua persons by reference to the common currency of the goals of the individual.

5. Joseph Raz (1997) denied that there are "brute wants"; instead, he argued, "There is always a reason for any desire" (118).

6. For a more literal type of "infinitism" in the realm of epistemology, see Klein 1999.

7. Another issue is how to compare health status from person to person, or even of the same person at different times:

"If two situations involve different preferences there is no standard of comparison on the basis of which these two situations can be compared. Therefore, it does not make sense to rate one's well-being in a possible situation where one's preferences have changed. Let us call this conclusion the *incommensurability thesis*" (Sandøe and Kappel 1994, 176).

8. For a related discussion, see Brock and Wartman 1990.

9. Mark Amadeus Notturno was helpful by highlighting this issue in conversation.

10. According to deontological ethical theories, the moral value of an action depends on what kind of action it is rather than on any consequences that follow from it.

11. According to consequentialist ethical theories, the moral value of an action depends not on what kind of action it is but rather on its consequences.

12. "One aspect of respecting persons is respecting their autonomy; this is an implication of respecting persons as independent ends in themselves" (Childress 1982, 59).

13. "... the reality of health is consistent with there being some conventional (nonrealistic) differences in what is considered a healthy person. Underlying these differences are standards of health that can only be accounted for by realism. But we must not assume that these standards are some sort of absolute standard" (Bloomfield 2001, 35).

Chapter 6

1. A version of this chapter was presented at Lafayette College in March 2002. I am grateful for helpful comments from George Panichas and his colleagues.

2. "Philosophers and others favoring the advance directive approach ['to determining how aggressively to treat seriously ill incompetent patients'] have contended that since autonomy is and ought to be assigned a high priority by most members of this society, it should carry the most weight in resolving decisions on medical treatment" (Dresser 1994, S2).

3. Advance directive brochures were procured from five hospitals in three eastern Pennsylvania health care systems in 2002. They all used the exact same text for the sample living will.

4. "(A) EXECUTION.—An individual of sound mind who is 18 years of age or older or who has graduated from high school or has married may execute at any time a declaration governing the initiation, continuation, withholding or withdrawal of life-sustaining treatment. The declaration must be signed by the declarant, or by another on behalf of and at the direction of the declarant, and must be witnessed by two individuals each of whom is 18 years of age or older. A witness shall not be the person who signed the declaration on behalf of and at the direction of the declarant" (Pennsylvania Consolidated Statutes 2002).

5. Sugarman (1994) made a similar point:

"While related work regarding preferences for other medical therapies (such as analgesia during labor and delivery) suggests that preferences are more stable if individuals have previously experienced the condition for which the therapy is indicated, it seems difficult to simulate the experience of a condition requiring life-sustaining treatment" (S12).

In consideration of this, Peter A. Singer (1994) discussed "disease-specific advance directives" for patients already suffering from a particular condition and who may thus already identify as someone facing the relevant issues.

6. "To date, three empirical studies have found that the presence of a formal advance directive had no significant effect on the end-of-life care subjects received" (Dresser 1994, S3).

7. Emanuel and Emanuel (1993) promoted a communitarian view of autonomy (or what serves for the communitarian as the analogue of autonomy). The theory holds:

". . . that ethical problems can be resolved only by accepting a public conception of the good life, while rejecting the conception of the good particular to utilitarianism. The idea is to move from individual consent to what some have called "informed community consent" by granting local communities the ethical and political authority to articulate and to enact their own conception of the good" (Emanuel 1987, 18).

8. A similar but less comprehensive advance directive document was used for an empirical study of the stability of treatment preferences. It describes three situations and four treatment options (CPR, mechanical breathing, artificial nutrition and hydration, and antibiotics). The instrument allows patients to specify that they want, do not want, or are undecided about each option in each case. (Kohut et al. 1997, 133–34)

9. D. Doukas shared some of this lineage in conversation.

10. I think it important to ascertain the patient's values with respect to distributive justice, as well as other values. Individuals might be upset to know that resources were used on them that could have been used to greater effect to help someone else.

11. For reasons unknown, this booklet is no longer available on their Web site.

12. The statute continues:

"(B) EMPLOYEE OR STAFF MEMBER OF HEALTH CARE PROVIDER.— An employee or staff member of a health care provider shall not be required to participate in the withholding or withdrawal of life-sustaining treatment. It shall be unlawful for an employer to discharge or in any other manner to discriminate against an employee or staff member who informs the employer that he does not wish to participate in the withholding or withdrawal of life-sustaining treatment."

13. Although accepting competition between autonomy and beneficence, Marion Danis (1994) made a similar point:

"For the purposes of following an advance directive, futility should be defined according to the patient's goals. . . . if the physician and patient agree upon the goals, but the physician does not believe it is possible to achieve them, despite apparent inconsistency with an advance directive, treatment may be withheld" (S22).

The Emanuels' medical directive has a loophole for futile treatments:

". . . the patient's right to refuse treatment does not imply a right to demand any intervention. In particular, a patient does not have the right to demand interventions that the physician considers futile. Recognizing this important point, the Medical Directive makes all requests for treatments conditional, stating in each scenario that requests apply only 'if considered medically reasonable'" (Emanuel and Emanuel 1989, 3292).

Note, however, the way that this wording suggests a separation between medical reasons (what is medically reasonable) and reasons based on autonomy. As I stated in part II, my concept of health qua person suggests that these two are more intimately connected.

14. "It is worth pointing out that the current practice with respect to advance directives does *not* recognize the right of an individual to bind his or her *competent* self in the future" (Buchanan and Brock 1989, 171–72).

15. The relevant issues can also be generated by thinking of the change in terms of discontinuity in the life narrative:

"When a person is radically changed and the narrative theme of this person's life–the theme that motivated the advance directive–has changed, the advance directive may no longer be valid. Although it is in practice extremely difficult, first, to define clearly which people belong in this liminal category and second, to know their wishes, it may occasionally be reasonable to disregard their advance directives. People have a surviving interest in managing their moments of incapacity, but people also have an interest in being protected from unreasonable bondage to an action they would have changed if they could" (Emanuel 1994, S27).

16. ". . . even where diminution of psychological continuity is great enough to lead us to conclude that the incompetent individual is not the person who issued the advance directive, we might nevertheless conclude that there is enough psychological continuity to give the wishes expressed in the advance directive *some weight* in our decision concerning the treatment of the incompetent individual" (Buchanan and Brock 1989, 183).

17. ". . . suppose an individual undergoes a significant change in circumstances during the time between executing the directive and becoming incapacitated by illness or injury. Might certain alterations create the possibility that a new individual has emerged?" (Dresser 1989, 157–58).

18. Cf., e.g., Danis 1994.

Chapter 7

1. Robert M. Veatch has argued along these lines.

2. For an interesting early discussion, see Szasz and Hollender 1956.

3. "In both medical emergencies and cases in which a serious condition has been diagnosed, which will require a series of treatments with significant side effects,

the provision of information and alternatives *may* enhance autonomous choice, but the provision of extensive information and alternatives, without some other form of support in decision making, may impede a person's decision-making capacity" (Dodds 2000, 231).

4. "In health matters, there will rarely be a single best answer on which the physician is the expert. He or she is the unquestioned expert on pathophysiological probabilities, but a medical decision involves deciding how much pain matters, whether a longer life is a good thing, and what kind of risk is bearable. On these, the physician is no expert, except perhaps for what he or she has learned from other patients' lives" (Andre 1992, 1411).

5. "These descriptions apply to communication behaviors used when the medical history is taken, but are considered to be representative of communication at other stages of the clinical encounter, as well" (Stewart 1995).

6. Ong et al. (1995) cast some doubt on this.

7. Cole and Bird (2000) remark:

"Interview training programs in medical schools have undergone significant evolution in recent years. Previously, many of these courses were focused on 'history taking' as the principal goal of the communication process—that is, on only one of the three core functions of the interview" (3).

8. Cole and Bird (2000) offer a thoughtful table linking the three functions to the objectives to be reached in implementing each function and the skills necessary to implement each well (281–82).

9. "There can be a tension between the needs of the clinician, the needs of the institution, and the needs of the patient and their family. . . . If you think through your goals prior to the interview, it will be easier during the interview to establish a healthy balance between your needs and the patient's" (Bickley and Hoekelman 1999, 4–5).

10. Outside the textbook literature, Calman's theory of quality of life can be applied in four stages. These stages could as well be tasks of a medical interview designed to address health of the patient qua person:

(i) Assessment. The patient's own list of problems and priorities, the estimation of the 'gap' [between goals and reality].

(ii) Development of a plan for modification of quality of life, with full involvement of the patient.

(iii) Implementation of the actions identified to meet the specific needs.

(iv) Evaluation of the outcome of the intervention and a review of the goals set. (Calman 1984, 127)

11. Orient (2000) warns against "misuse" of this question: "Instead of using it to encourage the patient to talk, some were using it defensively to get the patient to stop talking about problems that did not interest the doctors" (18).

12. *Bates' Guide* identifies six domains relevant to patient-centered care:

1. The patient's thoughts about the nature and the cause of the problem

2. The patient's feelings about the problem, especially fears

3. The patient's expectations of the clinician and health care

4. The effect of the problem on the patient's life

5. Similar experiences in the patient's personal or family history

6. Any steps that the patient has taken to address the problem (Bickley and Hoekelman 1999, 10)

13. Outside of the textbook literature, Ganzini et al. (1993) connected patient-centered care with informed consent:

"In order to give informed consent to accept or refuse medical treatment, a patient must be able to understand information about the procedure, appreciate the implications of the illness and the expected outcomes of treatment in terms of his other values and life goals, manipulate this information rationally, and communicate a stable treatment choice" (47).

14. *Bates' Guide* embraces this distinction between disease as biological explanation of symptoms and illness as patient experience of symptoms (Bickley and Hoekelman 1999, 10).

15. Hellström et al. describe a man who was intent on having doctors confirm with diagnosis his sense of being physically ill. The patient seemed to have been kept from leading a normal life by dissatisfaction with his medical interactions. They suggest that the patient's life might have been more healthy and satisfying if the physicians he consulted had been more attuned to his need for dialogue (Hellström, Lindqvist, and Mattsson 1998).

16. "Practioners . . . need the skills to provide clients with support and an opportunity to discharge their pain and distress, so that they can make the momentous and often painful decisions with which they are faced. It is only when practitioners are themselves able to do this, or see that it is adequately done by others, that medical knowledge will be correctly applied, that is, applied in a way that promotes and enhances people's health" (Whitbeck 1981b, 624).

17. ". . . the entire story as seen from the Patient's perspective has nothing whatsoever to do with his opinion of green eggs and ham (remember, he has never tasted them), but has *everything* to do with his relationship—or lack thereof—with the person who is offering them to him" (Forrow 1994, S31).

18. Forrow's discussion of the question *why?* makes a parallel point:

"In trying to understand and further explore any preference expressed by a patient, there is one simple question that is more important than any other: Why? An understanding of why a patient is expressing a particular preference is likely to give us much more solid guidance about that patient's own values and goals—and the ways in which the expressed preference may or may not represent them—than any number of invitations to the patient to reaffirm (or revise) that preference" (Forrow 1994, S31).

19. "We need to learn, first, how best to help individuals develop (discover?) and articulate 'authentic' preferences about what goals of care are most important to them; and, second, how to engage as clinicians in conversations with them that yield confirmation that those apparent preferences *are* 'authentic' and *do* reflect important values" (Forrow 1994, S31).

20. "*Tekné* here means a knowledge of how to act according to what is the case and why it is the case" (Pellegrino and Thomasma 1981, 69).

21. I make a parallel point about scientific research and research ethics (Richman 2002).

Chapter 8

1. Charles Fried (1974) put these ideas together quite nicely:

"The ideal of human life to which the physician ministers is an ideal of a life fully, lucidly lived, a life whose major events and constraints are accepted and internalized into the structure that a free and thinking man creates of that life. And thus the experiences of illness, cure and impending death must also be made into significant events that have intrinsic value. Since the physician is deeply implicated in all of these events, however, and since he therefore encounters his patient at the *cruces* of his life, it is essential that this encounter be a social encounter out of whose human and social reality the most can be made" (99–100).

References

"ACGME Outcome Project." In Accreditation Council for Graduate Medical Education Web site. <http://www.acgme.org/outcome/comp/compMin.asp>. Accessed 28 September 1999.

American Medical Association. "Shape Your Health Care Future with Health Care Advance Directives." <http://www.ama-assn.org/public/booklets/lvgwill.htm>. Accessed 29 January 2002.

Americans with Disabilities Act, U.S. Code 42 (1990), §1201 et seq.

Andre, Judith. Letter re: *Models of the Physician-Patient Relationship*, by Ezekiel J. Emanuel and Linda L. Emanuel. *Journal of the American Medical Association* 268, no. 11 (1992): 1411–12.

Aristotle. *The Basic Works of Aristotle*, edited by Richard McKeon. New York: Random House, 1941.

Ashraf, Haroon. "Surgery Offers Little Help for Patients with Body Dysmorphic Disorder." *Lancet* 355, no. 9220 (2000): 2055.

Audi, Robert. "Contemporary Foundationalism." In *The Theory of Knowledge: Classical and Contemporary Readings*, edited by Louis P. Pojman. Second edition, 204–11. Belmont, CA: Wadsworth Publishing Company, 1998.

Basmajian, John V. and Charles E. Slonecker. *Grant's Method of Anatomy: A Clinical Problem-Solving Approach*. Eleventh edition. Baltimore: Williams & Wilkins, 1989.

BBC News. "Woman Welcomes 'Right to Die' Ruling." In BBCi. <http://news.bbc.co.uk/hi/english/health/newsid_1887000/1887281.stm>. Accessed 23 March 2002.

Beauchamp, Tom L. and James F. Childress. *Principles of Biomedical Ethics*. Fifth edition. New York: Oxford University Press, 2001.

Beck, Aaron T. and Ruth L. Greenberg. "Brief Cognitive Therapies." In *Essential Papers on Short-Term Dynamic Therapy*, edited by James E. Groves, 230–47. New York: New York University Press, 1996.

Beck, Aaron T. et al. *Cognitive Therapy of Depression*. New York: Guilford Press, 1979.

Bertakis, Klea D., Debra Roter, and Samuel M. Putnam. "The Relationship of Physician Medical Interview Style to Patient Satisfaction." *Journal of Family Practice* 32, no. 2 (1991): 175–81.

Bickley, Lynn S. and Robert A. Hoekelman, with Elizabeth H. Naumburg and Joyce Beebe Thompson. *Bates' Guide to Physical Examination and History Taking*. Seventh edition. Philadelphia: J. B. Lippincott, 1999.

Billings, J. Andrew and John D. Stoeckle. *The Clinical Encounter: A Guide to the Medical Interview and Case Presentation*. Chicago: Year Book Medical Publishers, 1989.

Bloomfield, Paul. *Moral Reality*. New York: Oxford University Press, 2001.

Boorse, Christopher. "On the Distinction Between Disease and Illness." *Philosophy and Public Affairs* 5 (1975): 49–68.

———. "Health as a Theoretical Concept." *Philosophy of Science* 44 (1977): 542–73.

Brandt, Richard B. *A Theory of the Good and the Right*. Oxford: Oxford University Press, 1979.

Brock, Dan W. and Steven A. Wartman. "When Competent Patients Make Irrational Choices." *New England Journal of Medicine* 322, no. 22 (1990): 1595–99.

Brody, Howard. "Transparency: Informed Consent in Primary Care." *Hastings Center Report* 19 (1989): 5–9.

———. *The Healer's Power*. New Haven, CT: Yale University Press, 1992.

Buchanan, Allen E. and Dan W. Brock. *Deciding for Others: The Ethics of Surrogate Decisionmaking*. New York: Cambridge University Press, 1989.

Buchanan, Allen et al. *From Chance to Choice: Genetics and Justice*. Cambridge: Cambridge University Press, 2000.

Buford, Bill. "Delta Nights: A Singer's Love Affair with the Blues." *New Yorker*, 5 June 2000, 50–65.

Burgess, Michael et al. "Pediatric Care: Judgements about Best Interests at the Onset of Life." In *A Cross-Cultural Dialogue on Health Care Ethics*, edited by Harold Coward and Pinit Ratanakul, 160–75. Waterloo, ON: Wilfrid Laurier University Press, 1999.

Calman, K. C. "Quality of Life in Cancer Patients—An Hypothesis." *Journal of Medical Ethics* 10 (1984): 124–27.

Campbell, Margaret L. "Interpretation of an Ambiguous Advance Directive." *Dimensions of Critical Care Nursing* 14, no. 5 (1995): 226–32.

Caplan, Arthur L. "The Concepts of Health, Illness, and Disease." In *Companion Encyclopedia of the History of Medicine*, edited by W. Bynum and Roy Porter, vol. I, 233–48. London: Routledge, 1993.

Cassell, E. J. "The Function of Medicine." *Hastings Center Report* 7, no. 7 (1977): 16–19.

Chang, Ruth. "Introduction." In *Incommensurability, Incomparability, and Practical Reason*, edited by Ruth Chang, 1–34. Cambridge, MA: Harvard University Press, 1997.

Childress, James F. *Who Should Decide? Paternalism in Health Care*. New York: Oxford University Press, 1982.

Clayton, Matthew. Review of *Talking about Health: A Philosophical Dialogue*, by Lennart Nordenfelt (Atlanta: Rodolpi, 1997). *Journal of Medical Ethics* 25 (1999): 63.

Code, Lorraine. "Imagining Oneself Otherwise." In *Relational Autonomy: Feminist Perspectives on Autonomy, Agency, and the Social Self*, edited by Catriona Mackenzie and Natalie Stoljar, 124–50. New York: Oxford University Press, 2000.

Cohon, Rachel. "The Roots of Reasons." *Philosophical Review* 109, no. 1 (2000): 63–85.

Cole, Steven A. and Julian Bird. *The Medical Interview: The Three-Function Approach*. Second edition. Philadelphia: Mosby, 2000.

Coppola, Kristen M. et al. "Accuracy of Primary Care and Hospital-Based Physicians' Predictions of Elderly Outpatients' Treatment Preferences with and Without Advance Directives." *Archives of Internal Medicine* 161 (12 February 2001): 431–40.

Culver, C. M. and Bernard Gert. *Philosophy in Medicine: Conceptual and Ethical Issues in Medicine and Psychiatry*. New York: Oxford University Press, 1982.

Cummins, Robert. "Functional Analysis." In *Nature's Purposes: Analyses of Function and Design in Biology*, edited by Colin Allen, Marc Bekoff, and George Lauder, 169–96. Cambridge, MA: MIT Press, 1993.

Danis, Marion. "Following Advance Directives." *Hastings Center Report* 24, no. 6 (1994): S21–S23.

Davidson, Donald. "Mental Events." In *Essays on Actions and Events*, 207–27. Oxford: Oxford University Press, 1980.

———. "Radical Interpretation." In *Inquiries Into Truth and Interpretation*, 125–39. Oxford: Clarendon Press, 1984.

Davis, Daniel. "Phronesis, Clinical Reasoning, and Pellegrino's Philosophy of Medicine." *Theoretical Medicine* 18, no. 1–2 (1997): 173–95.

Dennett, Daniel C. *The Intentional Stance*. Cambridge, MA: MIT Press, 1987.

———. "Real Patterns." *Journal of Philosophy* LXXXVII (1991): 27–51.

Diagnostic and Statistical Manual of Mental Disorders. Fourth edition, text revision. Washington, DC: American Psychiatric Association, 2000.

Ditto, Peter H. et al. "Advance Directives as Acts of Communication: A Randomized Controlled Trial." *Archives of Internal Medicine* 161 (12 February 2001): 421–30.

Dodds, Susan. "Choice and Control in Feminist Bioethics." In *Relational Autonomy: Feminist Perspectives on Autonomy, Agency, and the Social Self*, edited by

Catriona Mackenzie and Natalie Stoljar, 213–35. New York: Oxford University Press, 2000.

Doukas, David. "Progress Report: The Task Force on Graduate Medical Education in Bioethics and the Humanities." Presented at the fifth annual meeting of the American Society for Bioethics and Humanities, Baltimore, MD, October 24–27, 2002.

Doukas, David J. and Laurence B. McCullough. "The Values History: The Evaluation of the Patient's Values and Advance Directives." *Journal of Family Practice* 32, no. 2 (1991): 145–54.

Drane, James F. "Competency to Give an Informed Consent: A Model for Making Clinical Assessments." *Journal of the American Medical Association* 252, no. 7 (1984): 925–27.

Dresser, Rebecca S. "Advance Directives, Self-Determination, and Personal Identity." In *Advance Directives in Medicine*, edited by Chris Hackler, Ray Mosely, and Dorothy E. Vawter, 155–70. New York: Praeger, 1989.

———. "Advance Directives: Implications for Policy." *Hastings Center Report* 24, no. 6 (1994): S2–S5.

Elliott, Carl. "A New Way to Be Mad." *Atlantic Monthly*, December 2000, 72–84.

Emanuel, Ezekiel J. "A Communal Vision of Care for Incompetent Patients." *Hastings Center Report* 17, no. 5 (1987): 15–20.

Emanuel, Ezekiel J. and Linda L. Emanuel. "Four Models of the Physician-Patient Relationship." *Journal of the American Medical Association* 267, no. 16 (1992): 2221–26.

Emanuel, Ezekiel J. et al. "How Well Is the Patient Self-Determination Act Working?: An Early Assessment." *American Journal of Medicine* 95, no. 6 (1993): 619–28.

Emanuel, Linda L. "What Makes a Directive Valid?" *Hastings Center Report* 24, no. 6 (1994): S27–29.

Emanuel, Linda L. and Ezekiel J. Emanuel. "The Medical Directive: A New Comprehensive Advance Care Document." *Journal of the American Medical Association* 261, no. 22 (1989): 3288–93.

———. "Decisions at the End of Life: Guided by Communities of Patients." *Hastings Center Report* 23, no. 5 (1993): 6–14.

Emanuel, Linda L. et al. "Advance Directives: Stability of Patients' Treatment Choices." *Archives of Internal Medicine* 154 (24 January 1994): 209–17.

Engelhardt Jr., H. Tristram. *The Foundations of Bioethics*. Second edition. New York: Oxford University Press, 1996.

Feldman, Mitchell D. and John F. Christensen. *Behavioral Medicine in Primary Care: A Practical Guide*. First edition. New York: Lange Medical Books/ McGraw-Hill, 1997.

Fodor, Jerry A. "Special Sciences." In *Representations: Philosophical Essays on the Foundations of Cognitive Science*, 127–45. Cambridge, MA: MIT Press, 1981.

———. "You Can Fool Some of the People All of the Time, Everything Else Being Equal; Hedged Laws and Psychological Explanations." *Mind* 100, no. 397 (1991): 19–34.

Forrow, Lachlan. "The Green Eggs and Ham Phenomena." *Hastings Center Report* 24, no. 6 (1994): S29–S32.

Frankena, William K. *Ethics*. Second edition. Englewood Cliffs, NJ: Prentice Hall, 1973.

Fried, Charles. *Medical Experimentation: Personal Integrity and Social Policy*. New York: American Elsevier, 1974.

Fukuyama, Francis. *Our Posthuman Future: Consequences of the Biotechnology Revolution*. New York: Farrar, Straus & Giroux, 2002.

Fulford, K. W. M. *Moral Theory and Medical Practice*. New York: Cambridge University Press, 1989.

Ganzini, Linda and Melinda A. Lee. "Authenticity, Autonomy, and Mental Disorders." *Journal of Clinical Ethics* 4, no. 1 (1993): 58–61.

Ganzini, Linda et al. "Is the Patient Self-Determination Act Appropriate for Elderly Persons Hospitalized for Depression?" *Journal of Clinical Ethics* 4, no. 1 (1993): 46–50.

Gawande, Atul. "Whose Body Is It, Anyway?: What Doctors Should Do when Patients Make bad Decisions." *New Yorker*, 4 October 1999, 85–91.

Geremia, Gina Marie. "Cognitive Therapy in the Treatment of Body Dysmorphic Disorder." Ph. D. dissertation, Hofstra University, 1998.

Giere, R. N. "Scientific Rationality as Instrumental Rationality." *Studies in the History and Philosophy of Science* 20 (1989): 377–84.

Gilligan, Carol. *In a Different Voice: Psychological Theory and Women's Development*. Cambridge, MA: Harvard University Press, 1982.

Gorbatenko-Roth, Kristina G. et al. "Accuracy of Health-Related Quality of Life Assessment: What Is the Benefit of Incorporating Patients' Preferences for Domain Functioning?" *Health Psychology* 20, no. 2 (2001): 136–40.

Gray's Anatomy: The Anatomical Basis of Medicine and Surgery, edited by Peter L. Williams. Thirty-eighth edition. New York: Churchill Livingstone, 1995.

Greenfield, Sheldon, Sherrie H. Kaplan, and John E. Ware Jr. "Expanding Patient Involvement in Care: Effects on Patient Outcomes." *Annals of Internal Medicine* 102, no. 4 (1985): 520–28.

Grisso, Thomas and Paul S. Appelbaum. *Assessing Competence to Consent to Treatment: A Guide for Physicians and Other Health Professionals*. New York: Oxford University Press, 1998.

Gunderman, Richard. "Illness as Failure: Blaming Patients." *Hastings Center Report* 30, no. 4 (2000): 7–11.

Hanson, Mark J. and Daniel Callahan. "Introduction." In *The Goals of Medicine: The Forgotten Issue in Health Care Reform*, edited by Mark J. Hanson and Daniel Callahan, ix–xiv. Washington, DC: Georgetown University Press, 1999.

Hare, R. M. *Moral Thinking: Its Levels, Method and Point.* Oxford: Oxford University Press, 1981.

Hastings Center. "Project Report: The Goals of Medicine: Setting New Priorities." In *The Goals of Medicine: The Forgotten Issue in Health Care Reform*, edited by Mark J. Hanson and Daniel Callahan, 1–54. Washington, DC: Georgetown University Press, 1999.

Häyry, Matti. "Measuring the Quality of Life: Why, How and What?" *Theoretical Medicine* 12 (1991): 97–116.

Hellström, O., P. Lindqvist, and B. Mattsson. "A Phenomenological Analysis of Doctor-Patient Interaction: A Case Study." *Patient Education and Counseling* 33 (1998): 83–89.

Helman, Cecil G. "Disease versus Illness in General Practice." *Journal of the Royal College of General Practitioners* 31 (1981): 548–52.

Herman, Barbara. "Mutual Aid and Respect for Persons." *Ethics* 94 (July 1984): 577–602.

Highfield, Roger. "Sufferers of Body Image Disorder Use DIY Surgery." *The Daily Telegraph* (London), 1 June 2000, Issue 1833, UK News.

Hitt, Jack. "The Year in Ideas: A to Z; Evidence-Based Medicine." *New York Times*, 9 December 2001, Sunday Magazine: 68.

Holden, C. "Random Samples." *Science* 285 (1999): 1007.

Hope, Tony, K. W. M. Fulford, and Anne Yates. *The Oxford Practice Skills Course: Ethics, Law, and Communication Skills in Health Care Education.* Oxford: Oxford University Press, 1996.

Hume, David. *A Treatise of Human Nature.* 1739–1740, edited by L. A. Selby-Bigge and P. H. Nidditch. Second edition. Oxford: Clarendon Press, 1978.

"Innovative Therapies Offer Hope for Young Cancer Patients." *Physicians Practice (Partners Healthcare Edition)* 10, no. 5 (2000): A2–A4.

Jones, Kenneth Lyons. *Smith's Recognizable Patterns of Human Malformation.* Fifth edition. Philadelphia: W. B. Saunders, 1997.

Jonsen, Albert R. "Casuistry." In *Encyclopedia of Bioethics*, edited by Warren T. Reich. Revised edition, vol. 1, 344–50. New York: Simon & Schuster Macmillan, 1995.

Jonsen, Albert R. and Stephen E. Toulmin. *The Abuse of Casuistry.* Berkeley: University of California Press, 1988.

Kant, Immanuel. *Foundations of the Metaphysics of Morals.* 1785. Translated by Lewis White Beck. Indianapolis: Bobbs-Merrill, 1959.

Kaplan, Sherrie H., Sheldon Greenfield, and John E. Ware Jr. "Assessing the Effects of Physician-Patient Interactions on the Outcomes of Chronic Disease." *Medical Care* 27, no. 3 Supplement (1989): S110–S127.

Klein, Peter D. "Human Knowledge and the Infinite Regress of Reasons." In *Philosophical Perspectives 13*, edited by James E. Tomberlin. Cambridge, MA: Blackwell, 1999.

Koggel, Christine M. *Perspectives on Equality: Constructing a Relational Theory*. Lanham, MD: Rowman & Littlefield, 1998.

Kohut, Nitsa et al. "Stability of Treatment Preferences: Although Most Preferences Do Not Change, Most People Change Some of Their Preferences." *Journal of Clinical Ethics* 8, no. 2 (1997): 124–35.

Korsgaard, Christine M. *Creating the Kingdom of Ends*. Cambridge: Cambridge University Press, 1996a.

———. *The Sources of Normativity*. Cambridge: Cambridge University Press, 1996b.

Kuhn, Thomas S. *The Structure of Scientific Revolutions*. Chicago: University of Chicago Press, 1962.

Lau, R. R., K. A. Hartman, and J. E. Ware Jr. "Health as a Value: Methodological and Theoretical Considerations." *Health Psychology* 5, no. 1 (1986): 25–43.

Laudan, Larry. "Normative Naturalism." *Philosophy of Science* 57 (1990): 44–59.

Lee, Melinda A. et al. "Do Patients' Treatment Decisions Match Advance Statements of Their Preferences?" *Journal of Clinical Ethics* 9, no. 3 (1998): 258–62.

Levi, Benjamin H. *Respecting Patient Autonomy*. Urbana: University of Illinois Press, 1999.

Lipkin Jr., Mack. "The Medical Interview." In *Behavioral Medicine in Primary Care: A Practical Guide*, edited by Mitchell D. Feldman and John F. Christensen, 1–7. New York: Lange Medical Books/McGraw-Hill, 1997.

Mackenzie, Catriona and Natalie Stoljar. "Introduction: Autonomy Refigured." In *Relational Autonomy: Feminist Perspectives on Autonomy, Agency, and the Social Self*, edited by Catriona Mackenzie and Natalie Stoljar, 3–31. New York: Oxford University Press, 2000.

Malebranche, Nicolas. *The Search after Truth*. 1674. Translated by Thomas M. Lennon and Paul J. Olscamp. Translation of the sixth edition. New York: Cambridge University Press, 1997.

McDowell, Ian and Claire Newell. *Measuring Health: A Guide to Rating Scales and Questionnaires*. Second edition. Oxford: Oxford University Press, 1996.

McGee, Glenn. "Phronesis in Clinical Ethics." *Theoretical Medicine* 17, no. 4 (1996): 317–28.

McMullin, Ernan. "Underdetermination." *Journal of Medicine and Philosophy* 20 (1995): 233–52.

Miller, Bruce. "Autonomy." In *Encyclopedia of Bioethics*, edited by Warren T. Reich. Revised edition, vol. 1, 215–20. New York: Simon & Schuster Macmillan, 1995.

Millgram, Elijah. "Incommensurability and Practical Reasoning." In *Incommensurability, Imcomparability, and Practical Reason*, edited by Ruth Chang, 151–69. Cambridge, MA: Harvard University Press, 1997.

Millikan, Ruth Garrett. *Language, Thought, and Other Biological Categories: New Foundations for Realism.* Cambridge, MA: MIT Press, 1984.

Mordacci, R. and R. Sobel. "Health: A Comprehensive Concept." *Hastings Center Report* 28, no. 1 (1998): 34–37.

Munson, Ronald. *Intervention and Reflection: Basic Issues in Medical Ethics.* Sixth edition. Belmont, CA: Wadsworth, 2000.

Nagel, Ernest. "Teleology Revisited." In *Nature's Purposes: Analyses of Function and Design in Biology*, edited by Colin Allen, Marc Bekoff, and George Lauder, 197–240. Cambridge, MA: MIT Press, 1998.

Nisbett, Richard E. and Lee Ross. *Human Inference: Strategies and Shortcomings of Social Judgment.* Englewood Cliffs, NJ: Prentice Hall, 1980.

Nordenfelt, Lennart. "Concepts of Health and Their Consequences for Health Care." *Theoretical Medicine* 14 (1993a): 277–85.

———. "On the Relation Between Biological and Social Theories of Health: A Commentary on Fulford's Praxis Makes Perfect." *Theoretical Medicine* 14 (1993b): 321–24.

———. "Mild Mania and the Theory of Health: A Response to 'Mild Mania and Well-Being.'" *Philosophy, Psychiatry and Psychology* 1, no. 3 (1994a): 179–84.

———. "Towards a Theory of Happiness: A Subjectivist Notion of Quality of Life." In *Concepts and Measurement of Quality of Life in Health Care*, edited by Lennart Nordenfelt, 35–57. Dordrecht: Kluwer Academic Publishers, 1994b.

———. *On the Nature of Health: An Action-Theoretic Approach.* Second edition. Dordrecht: Kluwer Academic Publishers, 1995.

O'Neill, Onora. "Universal Laws and Ends-in-Themselves." *Monist* 72 (1989): 341–61.

Ong, L. M. L. et al. "Doctor-Patient Communication: A Review of the Literature." *Social Science and Medicine* 40, no. 7 (1995): 903–18.

Orient, Jane M. *Sapira's Art and Science of Bedside Diagnosis.* Second edition. Philadelphia: Lippincott Williams & Wilkins, 2000.

Ostenfeld, Erik. "Aristotle on the Good Life and Quality of Life." In *Concepts and Measurement of Quality of Life in Health Care*, edited by Lennart Nordenfelt, 19–34. Dordrecht: Kluwer Academic Publishers, 1994.

Oxford English Dictionary. Oxford University Press. <http://dictionary.oed.com/>. Accessed August 2001.

Parfit, Derek. *Reasons and Persons*. Oxford: Oxford University Press, 1984.

Patterson, Kevin. "What Doctors Don't Know (Almost Everything)." *New York Times*, 5 May 2002, Sunday Magazine: 74–77.

Pennsylvania Consolidated Statutes. *Title 20, Chapter 54: Advance Directive for Health Care* 5404 (2002).

Pellegrino, Edmund D. Review of *The Practice of Autonomy: Patients, Doctors and Medical Decisions*, by Carl E. Schneider. (New York: Oxford University Press, 1998). *Theoretical Medicine and Bioethics* 21 (2000): 361–65.

Pellegrino, Edmund D. and David C. Thomasma. *A Philosophical Basis of Medical Practice: Toward a Philosophy and Ethic of the Healing Professions*. New York: Oxford University Press, 1981.

———. *For the Patient's Good: The Restoration of Beneficence in Health Care*. New York: Oxford University Press, 1988.

Pörn, Ingmar. "An Equilibrium Model of Health." In *Health, Disease, and Causal Explanations in Medicine*, edited by L. Nordenfelt and B. I. B. Lindahl, 3–9. Boston: D. Reidel, 1984.

———. "Health and Adaptedness." *Theoretical Medicine* 14, no. 4 (1993): 295–303.

Putnam, Samuel M. et al. "Patient Exposition and Physician Explanation in Initial Medical Interviews and Outcomes of Clinic Visits." *Medical Care* 23, no. 1 (1985): 74–83.

Quine, W. V. O. "Reply to Morton White." In *The Philosophy of W. V. Quine*, edited by L. A. Hahn and P. A. Schilpp, 663–65. LaSalle, IL: Open Court, 1986.

Railton, Peter. "Moral Realism." *Philosophical Review* XCV, no. 2 (1986): 163–207.

Ramsay, Sarah. "Controversy Over UK Surgeon Who Amputated Healthy Limbs." *Lancet* 355, no. 9202 (2000): 476.

Rawls, John. *A Theory of Justice*. Cambridge, MA: Harvard University Press, 1971.

Raz, Joseph. "Incommensurability and Agency." In *Incommensurability, Incomparability, and Practical Reason*, edited by Ruth Chang, 110–28. Cambridge, MA: Harvard University Press, 1997.

Richman, Kenneth A. "Responsible Conduct of Research Is all Well and Good." *American Journal of Bioethics* 2, no. 4 (2002): 62–63.

Richman, Kenneth A. and Andrew E. Budson. "Health of Organisms and Health of Persons." Presented at the Pacific division meetings of the American Philosophical Association, Albuquerque, NM; April, 2000a.

———. "Health of Organisms and Health of Persons: An Embedded Instrumentalist Approach." *Theoretical Medicine and Bioethics* 21, no. 4 (2000b): 339–52.

Rockwood, Kenneth, Paul Stolee, and Roy A. Fox. "Use of Goal Attainment Scaling in Measuring Clinically Important Change in the Frail Elderly." *Journal of Clinical Epidemiology* 46, no. 10 (1993): 1113–18.

Roe v. Wade, 35 L.Ed.2d 147 (U.S. 1973).

Ross, Judith Wilson. "Practice Guidelines: Texts in Search of Authority." In *Getting Physicians to Listen: Ethics and Outcomes Data in Context*, edited by Philip J. Boyle, 41–70. Washington, DC: Georgetown University Press, 1998.

Ross, W. D. *The Right and the Good*. Oxford: Clarendon Press, 1930.

Rudwick, M. J. S. "The Inference of Function from Structure in Fossils." In *Nature's Purposes: Analyses of Function and Design in Biology*, edited by Colin Allen, Marc Bekoff, and George Lauder, 101–15. Cambridge, MA: MIT Press, 1998.

Sacks, Oliver. *The Man Who Mistook His Wife for a Hat*. New York: Harper & Row, 1970.

Sade, R. M. "A Theory of Health and Disease: The Objectivist-Subjectivist Dichotomy." *Journal of Medicine and Philosophy* 20 (1995): 513–25.

Sandøe, Peter. "Quality of Life—Three Competing Views." *Ethical Theory and Moral Practice* 2, no. 1 (1999): 11–23.

Sandøe, Peter and Klemens Kappel. "Changing Preferences: Conceptual Problems in Comparing Health-Related Quality of Life." In *Concepts and Measurement of Quality of Life in Health Care*, edited by L. Nordenfelt, 161–80. Dordrecht: Kluwer Academic Publishers, 1994.

Schneider, Carl E. *The Practice of Autonomy: Patients, Doctors and Medical Decisions*. New York: Oxford University Press, 1998.

Seedhouse, David. *Health: The Foundations for Achievement*. New York: John Wiley & Sons, 1986.

Seuss, Dr. (Theodor Seuss Geisel). *Green Eggs and Ham*. New York: Random House, 1960.

Shaw, Anthony. "Defining the Quality of Life." *Hastings Center Report* 7, no. 5 (1977): 11.

Siegel, Harvey. "Naturalism, Instrumental Rationality, and the Normativity of Epistemology." *Protosoz* 8/9 (1996): 97–110.

Siegler, Mark. "The Doctor-Patient Encounter and Its Relationship to Theories of Health and Disease." In *Concepts of Health and Disease: Interdisciplinary Perspectives*, edited by Arthur L. Caplan, H. Tristram Engelhardt Jr., and James J. McCartney, 627–44. Reading, MA: Addison-Wesley, 1981.

Singer, Peter A. "Disease-Specific Advance Directives." *Lancet* 344 (27 August 1994): 594–96.

Somerset, Maggie et al. "What Do People with MS Want and Expect from Health-Care Services?" *Health Expectations* 4, no. 1 (2001): 29–37.

Stewart, Moira A. "What Is a Successful Doctor-Patient Interview? A Study of Interactions and Outcomes." *Social Science and Medicine* 19, no. 2 (1984): 167–75.

————. "Effective Physician-Patient Communication and Health Outcomes: A Review." *Canadian Medical Association Journal* 152, no. 9 (1995): 1423–33.

Stewart, William. *Counselling in Rehabilitation*. London: Croom Helm, 1985.

Stich, Stephen P. "Dennett on Intentional Systems." *Philosophical Topics* 12 (1981): 39–62.

————. *The Fragmentation of Reason: Preface to a Pragmatic Theory of Cognitive Evaluation*. Cambridge, MA: MIT Press, 1990.

Stineman, Margaret G. "Defining the Population, Treatments, and Outcomes of Interest: Reconciling the Rules of Biology with Meaningfulness." *American Journal of Physical Medicine and Rehabilitation* 80, no. 2 (2001): 147–59.

Stineman, Margaret G. et al. "Comparing Consumer and Clinician Values for Alternative Functional States: Application of a New Feature Trade-off Consensus Building Tool." *Archives of Physical Medicine and Rehabilitation* 79 (December 1998): 1522–29.

Stone, Martin. "Casuistry." In *Routledge Encyclopedia of Philosophy*, edited by Edward Craig, vol. 2, 227–29. London: Routledge, 1998.

Stuttaford, Thomas. "A Craving for Change Can Be Obsessive." *Times* (London), 3 February 2000, Home News.

Sugarman, Jeremy. "Recognizing Good Decisionmaking for Incapacitated Patients." *Hastings Center Report* 24, no. 6 (1994): S11–S13.

Swanson, J. et al. "Acute Tolerance to Methylphenidate in the Treatment of Attention Deficit Hyperactivity Disorder in Children." *Clinical Pharmacology & Therapeutics* 66, no. 3 (1999): 295–305.

Swartz, Mark H. *Textbook of Physical Diagnosis: History and Examination*. Philadelphia: W. B. Saunders, 1989.

Szasz, Thomas S. "The Myth of Mental Illness." *American Psychologist* 15 (1960): 113–18.

————. "Second Commentary on 'Aristotle's Function Argument.'" *Philosophy, Psychiatry and Psychology* 7, no. 1 (2000): 3–16.

Szasz, Thomas S. and Marc H. Hollender. "The Basic Models of the Doctor-Patient Relationship." *Archives of Internal Medicine* 97 (1956): 585–92.

Tanenbaum, Sandra J. "Knowing and Acting in Medical Practice: The Epistemological Politics of Outcomes Research." In *Meaning and Medicine: A Reader in the Philosophy of Health Care*, edited by James Lindemann Nelson and Hilde Lindemann Nelson, 61–72. New York: Routledge, 1994.

Thagard, Paul. "Explaining Disease: Correlations, Causes and Mechanisms." In *Explanation and Cognition*, edited by Frank C. Keil and Robert A. Wilson, 254–76. Cambridge, MA: MIT Press, 2000.

Tversky, Amos and Daniel Kahneman. "Judgment Under Uncertainty." In *Judgment Under Uncertainty: Heuristics and Biases*, edited by Daniel Kahneman, Paul Slovic, and Amos Tversky, 3–20. New York: Cambridge University Press, 1982.

Unger, Peter K. *Identity, Consciousness, and Value*. New York: Oxford University Press, 1990.

Veatch, Robert M. "Models for Ethical Medicine in a Revolutionary Age: What Physician-Patient Roles Foster the Most Ethical Relationship?" *Hastings Center Report* 2, no. 3 (1972): 5–7.

Veatch, Robert M. and William E. Stempsey S. J. "Incommensurability: Its Implications for the Patient/Physician Relationship." *Journal of Medicine and Philosophy* 20, no. 3 (1995): 253–69.

Von Korff, Michael et al. "Collaborative Management of Chronic Illness." *Annals of Internal Medicine* 127, no. 12 (1997): 1097–102.

Wanzer, Sidney H. et al. "The Physician's Responsibility Toward Hopelessly Ill Patients. A Second Look." *New England Journal of Medicine* 320, no. 13 (1989): 844–49.

Wason, P. C. and P. N. Johnson-Laird. *Psychology of Reasoning: Structure and Content*. New York: Harvard University Press, 1972.

Whitbeck, Caroline. "On the Aims of Medicine: Comments on 'Philosophy of Medicine as the Source for Medical Ethics.'" *Metamedicine* 2 (1981a): 35–41.

———. "A Theory of Health." In *Concepts of Health and Disease: Interdisciplinary Perspectives*, edited by Arthur L. Caplan, H. Tristram Engelhardt Jr., and James J. McCartney, 611–26. Reading, MA: Addison-Wesley, 1981b.

Wiggins, David. "Incommensurability: Four Proposals." In *Incommensurability, Incomparability, and Practical Reason*, edited by Ruth Chang, 52–66. Cambridge, MA: Harvard University Press, 1997.

Williams, Patricia J. *The Alchemy of Race and Rights*. Cambridge, MA: Harvard University Press, 1991.

Wright, Larry. "Functions." In *Nature's Purposes: Analyses of Function and Design in Biology*, edited by Collin Allen, Marc Bekoff, and George Lauder, 51–78. Cambridge, MA: MIT Press, 1998.

Wulff, Henrik R. "The Inherent Paternalism in Clinical Practice." *Journal of Medicine and Philosophy* 20, no. 3 (1995): 299–311.

Index